DOUBLE
Your
Haircolor
Income
in 30 Days!

DOUBLE Your Haircolor Income in 30 Days!

MARK D. FOLEY

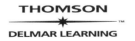

THOMSON

™

DELMAR LEARNING

Australia   Canada   Mexico   Singapore   Spain   United Kingdom   United States

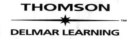

Double Your Haircolor Income in 30 Days!
Mark D. Foley

President:
Dawn Gerrain

Director of Production:
Wendy A. Troeger

Director of Marketing:
Wendy Mapstone

Director of Editorial:
Sherry Gomoll

Production Coordinator:
Nina Tucciarelli

Channel Manager:
Sandra Bruce

Acquisitions Editor:
Stephen Smith

Composition:
Larry O'Brien

Marketing Coordinator:
Kasmira Koniszewski

Editorial Assistant:
Courtney VanAuskas

Library of Congress Cataloging-in-Publication Data

Foley, Mark D.
   Double your haircolor income in 30 days / by Mark Foley.
      p. cm.
   Includes bibliographical references.
   ISBN 1-4018-4461-8
   1. Beauty shops--Management. 2. Beauty shops--Marketing. 3. Hair--Dyeing and bleaching. I. Title.
   TT965.F6497 2005
   646.7'2'068--dc22
                                    2004008126

NOTICE TO THE READER

CONTENTS

PREFACE

I n many ways I am a reporter. Owning and operating my own salons over the years has brought me ample good fortune. Learning from others has made this so. I have spent more than a decade studying haircolor marketing. I have interacted with over 50,000 salon and spa professionals on ways to improve the financial performance of their business practices. I have invested countless hours with haircolor manufacturing company executives and distribution professionals, and I have consulted with dozens of salon chain owners.

Through all this, I have used my powers of observation and insight to distill the best ideas and methods to grow haircolor income for the professional cosmetologist. As you read, you will come to know my opinion of what is the best and most efficient approach to growing your haircolor business. There are other approaches out there. Here, I present what I believe to be the best approach.

Communication with clients is going to be a big key to your success. Because I am a professional communicator, I intentionally propose dozens of words and phrases for you to use. You will find many passages in quotes. When you see those in the context of talking with clients, recognize that I am proposing a dialogue for you to use. I am providing you with specific words and phrases that I know are effective. I am trying to help you script yourself so that you can be prepared to interact effectively even in the most delicate situations. Use them and make them your own.

ABOUT THE AUTHOR

Mark D. Foley is considered by many to be the foremost motivational and business educator in the beauty business today as well as the most electrifying and dynamic seminar leader in the salon profession. His expertise in salon management, marketing, and customer service has won him clients representing a who's who of salon industry standouts.

Mark has written or been featured in articles by all the major salon industry trade magazines. He has personally trained more than 35,000 salon professionals internationally since 1990.

Mark's seminars "How to Double Your Haircolor Income . . . in 30 days or less!" and "How to Achieve Supernatural Salon Income" rank as all time best-selling programs in the beauty business.

From a career as a highly successful owner of salons in Canada, Mark focuses his attention on writing, consulting, and speaking to communicate strategies for maximizing salon income and profits. An Eagle Scout and a graduate of Fordham University in New York, Mark makes his home in Seattle, Washington.

Mark has been recognized with academic honors and awards from Harvard University, The University of Pennsylvania, New York University, UCLA, USC, as well as the U.S. and Canadian governments. He has been the United States National Public Speaking Champion, the recipient of "The Golden Scroll Award" from The American Academy of Achievement, and the recipient of "The George Washington Medal of Honor" from The Freedoms Foundation at Valley Forge.

ACKNOWLEDGMENTS

Don and Flonnie Westbrook are haircolor marketing geniuses. As owners and operators of the remarkable elon Salon in Marietta, Georgia, they have perfected the principles outlined in this series. In fact, these remarkable folks developed a very significant percentage of the tools and techniques I've related.

The Westbrooks have single-handedly revolutionized the art and practice of salon haircolor marketing for the entire industry. They have influenced my own thinking on this more than all other sources combined. Owners, stylists, and colorists who have benefited from this program owe a debt of gratitude to the Westbrooks.

Even more heartwarming are the openness and sharing of the Westbrooks. Practically all of the illustrations in these pages were provided courtesy of the Westbrooks. This willingness to share freely tells you something remarkable about the Westbrooks—it is their uncompromising dedication to the principle that fearless giving is the singular principle of success and happiness in life. I have tried my best to live up to their standard of contribution through these pages.

I would also like to acknowledge the contributions of the following reviewers:

Carole Eckstrom
Paragon Hair & Nails
Altamote Springs, FL

Kevin Krelic
John & Friends Hair Design
Indianapolis, IN

Dee Levin
Salon Norman-Dee
Philadelphia, PA

Linda Craig
Looking Good Hair & Nail Salon
Redding, CA

INTRODUCTION

Welcome to Real Prosperity!

Right now you are in the midst of the biggest financial opportunity the beauty business will see this generation! It's haircolor! And believe it, because a lot of money is going to be made very quickly and companies and designers are going to be able to position themselves for legendary levels of profitability the likes of which will not be visited again in our lifetimes.

Rejoice! This news is the most positive development that the salon industry could have wished for. Colorists, hair designers, and salon and spa owners now have the real opportunity to make more money, achieve greater status and recognition, and experience more professional and artistic fulfilment than ever before—all because of the remarkable transformational power of haircolor.

You want to make sure that you are in that number. In this book you will find exactly the information you need to move boldly and with confidence to capitalize on these rare circumstances.

Welcome to the Age of Haircolor!

The salon and spa industry has entered into what can be called the Age of Color. Previously in the Age of Retail, which dated from approximately 1970 to 1990, most of the innovations in the salon business were driven by the explosion of salon product retailing. The Age of Retail brought with it innovations in the layout of salons to accommodate home product sales. Display and merchandising in the salon transformed. The financial perspectives of the business changed. New demands and opportunities were given to salon workers. A whole new type of retail salon emerged. The beauty store business mushroomed and morphed. Much continues to happen as these trends mature.

In the Age of Color, supplying the skyrocketing demand for color products and services will be the driving force of innovation in the salon industry for the next generation, well into the twenty-first century.

Just as with retail, color—and, for this book's purposes, haircolor —is going to impact every segment of the business in ways never before imagined. It is already happening. Specialty retail products are already being developed for haircolor enhancement and home maintenance. The way the business is analyzed will focus more on the financial advantages of haircolor. New salon specialties will become more pronounced. The layout of salons will be transformed to accommodate haircolor departments. A new breed of color salon and color spa will emerge strongly. Much has and will continue to happen!

Our purpose here is to reveal some of the key opportunities you as a salon and spa professional will want to focus on during the Age of Color. You will gain fresh insights and make strategic breakthroughs so that you can take full financial advantage of the runaway haircolor trend that is being experienced in the profession right now!

In *Double Your Haircolor Income in 30 Days!*, you will:

1. enliven your awareness and consciousness about the professional haircolor opportunity.

2. discover how to market yourself as a top color practitioner.

3. find out how you can position your salon as the place for coloring in your community.

4. learn ways to entice more salon guests into professional haircoloring.

5. determine ways to convert home-color users into professional haircoloring.

6. master methods to upgrade your salon color clientele into more elaborate and costly color services.

It is all about how you can bring professional haircolor to market more effectively. It is about situating yourself to experience the highest level of income now available to the salon professional.

And *Double Your Haircolor Income in 30 Days!* is not just an empty title. Many colorists and salon practitioners who put this information into practice will be satisfied to see a several thousand dollar increase in their haircolor income each year. However, the ideas and strategies you will be exposed to are capable of creating a salon revenue stream of a million dollars or more a year, if that is what you aspire to. Because professional haircoloring is what you are about, shoot for the stars both artistically and financially.

"Hair colorists can now situate themselves as the top income earners and highest status practitioners in the profession."

Pablo Picasso, the most famous painter of the twentieth century, shared this: "My mother said to me, 'If you become a soldier, you'll be a general; if you become a monk, you'll end up as the Pope.' Instead, I became a painter and wound up as Picasso."

Why not *you* now?

The Age of Haircolor

his is a generation for haircolor! Never before have people enjoyed such high aspirations and expected so much from life. Scientists explore the galaxy and the atom in an effort to harness the forces of nature and exercise more control over human destiny. At least seven ideas can help the beauty industry come to a clear understanding of the remarkable professional opportunity that presents itself with haircolor.

This is what you will discover about the Age of Haircolor:

1. Key population demographics demand haircoloring.
2. Haircolor is now totally accepted by Western society.
3. Haircolor delivers genuine value and benefits.
4. Everyone has access to haircolor's mystique.
5. Haircolor is prestigious.
6. Haircolor promotes loyalty through all segments of the business of beauty.
7. Haircolor maximizes salon income as well as individual opportunity.

Key Population Demographics Demand Haircoloring

Demography is the study of vital population statistics like births, deaths, and population segmentation.

As we now enter the twenty-first century, the post–World War II generation—often referred to as the baby boomers—dominates the social, economic, cultural, and political theater in the Western world. It is the largest population group ever known in the Western hemisphere. Approximately 75,000,000 baby boomers are coming of age right now in the United States alone. Each minute, several people turn 50 in North America. Every hour, 300 or more people turn 50 in the United States and Canada—a trend that will continue past 2015.

The financial status of this segment of the population is the best ever from a commercial standpoint. This demographic group has already made more money than any generation in history. Now, as they enter their 50s, they have more disposable income than ever as their offspring leave home and they become empty nesters. Plus, as their parents pass away over the next decade or two, boomers will be the recipients of the greatest transfer of wealth that the world has ever seen through inheritance.

Psychography is the study of a population's personality and character—how people think and behave. Psychologically, the baby-boom generation is a natural for haircolor. This is the generation that has spent the last 30 years selling youthfulness to the rest of the world. They have always prized the idea of looking good and feeling good. They are a group that has had high aspirations. And, they have demonstrated that they fully expect to continue to look and feel good well into their golden years.

Haircolor is about holding on to youth. And, one thing that can be successfully controlled to withstand the aging process is haircolor. We can control haircolor! We have already seen a tremendous growth in haircolor purchasing by the postwar generation. The baby boomers have demonstrated clearly that they want haircolor and that they can afford it. The sales of both professional haircolor and home haircolor are booming. Haircolor is and will remain the fastest growing segment in the beauty business.

Two haircolor trends are actually taking place that benefit salons. First, a larger percentage of the population is coloring their hair. Second, a larger percentage of those coloring their hair are having it done professionally in the salon. So, not only is the pie itself getting bigger, but the professional slice of that pie is also getting considerably bigger. It is easy to predict that these megatrends will continue—this will not be a short-lived fad!

In the 1980s perhaps as few as 5 percent of female haircolor applications were performed in salons. (More about haircolor and the male population a little later.) As of this writing nearing the turn of the century, salon market penetration has increased to perhaps 25 percent of female haircolor applications, by some estimates. Plus, during that time more and more millions of women every year have been converted to coloring their hair. Bigger pie, bigger slice!

The year 1992 is regarded as the beginning of the Age of Color because 1992 was the year that haircolor surpassed permanent waving and relaxing services in dollar volume at salons. The next time you visit a beauty supply store, notice that more shelf space is devoted to color than to perms and relaxers. This is particularly remarkable when you consider that salons dominate the perming and relaxing markets. Somewhere around 95 percent of perming and relaxing services have

"The haircolor market is growing and the salon industry's market share is expanding at the same time—a double win for beauty professionals."

historically been performed in salons with very few being done at home. Visit your local drug store and see for yourself how much shelf space is devoted to home perming and relaxing products. Now, compare that to the ever-growing drug store shelf space being devoted to haircolor preparations. You'll immediately get a feel for what has been and is happening. Haircolor now dominates both the consumer and the professional markets.

So, there is a high and growing demand for haircolor in general and professional haircolor in particular. This is in an environment of a generally shrinking cosmetology workforce. Any economist will tell you that when high demand is accompanied by limited supply, prices increase. Due to the forces of supply and demand, the prices of professional haircoloring services should go up noticeably in the years ahead. Therefore, providers of professional haircolor services should find themselves in an increasingly lucrative pursuit.

Haircolor Is Now Totally Accepted by Western Society

Those of us with some mileage know that haircolor was not always totally accepted. There was a time when nice girls did not color their hair. It has taken a tremendous amount of advertising and promotion, funded by the major haircolor manufacturers, to turn that public attitude around. This has been at some great expense. Compare mass media advertising for haircoloring to that for permanent waving, for example, and it isn't even close! Relentless marketing has created popular acceptance of haircolor.

Granted, the very expensive high-quality haircolor advertising has been focused on promoting home coloring preparations available to the mass market. Nevertheless professional haircolor sales have benefited from the growing popular appeal prompted by this advertising.

There have been celebrity spokespersons for some time. The appeal of color advertising and promotion keeps improving. Haircoloring is being positioned as high fashion. It has taken on a more glamorous and fashionable aura than ever before. It's in all the magazines. It's on the talk shows. The top models wear it on the fashion runways. You name it, haircolor is there!

Exclusive professional brands will soon engage in even more mass media haircolor promotion. During the Age of Retail, big salon retail lines engaged in mass media promotions. This will happen with haircolor too.

The universal acceptance of haircolor in American culture has happened. The universal use of haircolor in American culture, on the other hand, has not yet happened. It is most reasonable to expect remarkable strides in converting more of the population to haircoloring in the years ahead.

This prediction is based on the phenomenon of herd mentality. Herd mentality is a well-known evolutionary experience in populations that was first noted by Charles Darwin. When Darwin studied the Rhesus Monkeys of the Galapagos Islands off South America, he discovered that a small group of them would use a peculiar sharp edged rock to easily open the shell of the nut that was their dietary staple. Even though the benefit of this technique was clear, it took considerable chattering and demonstration to convert each additional monkey to this method. But, one by one, the population of monkeys using the rock as a tool grew. Darwin observed that once the practice was accepted and used by a certain critical mass of the population, then herd mentality took over and suddenly the entire population adopted the practice at once. That threshold of critical mass Darwin called "The Hundredth Monkey." This predictable phenomenon has become known as "The Hundredth Monkey Principle."

It is the author's belief that we are on the threshold of critical mass with haircolor! The Hundredth Monkey Principle has paid frequent visits to the fashion and grooming world. Fashion and grooming are social practices, and as social animals humans have a powerful need for acceptance and even recognition. For example, when the herd mentality was that bell-bottom pants were out of fashion and no longer socially acceptable, the practice of wearing bell-bottom pants stopped promptly. The threat of being ostracized by the herd meant everyone conformed.

Just as people shampoo, condition, and comb or dress their hair as a standard course of action to appear acceptable in society, so too the population will wear color in their hair. It will just be what we do!

To some this may sound peculiar. But consider that only a few decades ago, the herd mentality compelled people in Western civilizations to universally adopt the practice of using deodorants and antiperspirants, which had just recently been invented. Funny as it may seem, body odor, which is part of the natural human condition, was deemed unacceptable by the herd. So too, the very strong perfumes that some wore were given thumbs down. If you wanted to be accepted, then body odor was no longer an option. The human need to be socially acceptable is so powerful that today the practice of including deodorants and antiperspirants as part of the personal hygiene regime is not even questioned. By today's standards, if you allow the natural state of body odor to linger about your person, many will consider you backward and it is most likely that you will be ridiculed and ostracized over it.

Could the same attitude develop regarding the natural state of gray hair? Imagine if naturally occurring gray hair was seen to be an indication of laziness and less than acceptable personal grooming (just the way naturally occurring body odor is perceived). If that were to happen, the human need to be accepted by society would surely compel the population to haircoloring. It is something to consider.

> **"Just as people shampoo their hair to appear well groomed, so too they will wear color in their hair. It will just be what we do!"**

Another example is that at the dawn of the Age of Retail, many patrons came to the salon having already shampooed their hair at home so that they did not have to spend the extra fifty cents to have it done at the salon. This was particularly true of male clients and nonweekly female visitors. Those who have been around a few years know that this was quite common. During the Age of Retail, salons were able to convert virtually all patrons to a professional shampoo and conditioning service, even though at one time many considered it too expensive, too luxurious, or too embarrassing. The following factors were key to this transformation:

- Salons began to package cutting services to include the shampoo.
- Salons energetically engaged in the merchandising, display, and promotion of professional salon products.
- Salons communicated with their clients.

There were several years of slow but sure progress. A lot of chattering and demonstration went on to convince more and more patrons to allow the professionals to shampoo their hair at the salon. Then, suddenly, practically without anyone taking notice, the entire population of salon patrons simply accepted the shampoo as part of the cutting service. Today, the shampoo is virtually automatic—the 100th monkey! The only exception may be some chain and franchised operations that use a low haircut lead-in price to build traffic among cost-conscious consumers. For that purpose these businesses maintain their à la carte pricing.

The day will come, before anyone realizes it, when a color or rinse or other brightening treatment will just be an automatic occurrence. It will be packaged right into the standard cutting service the way restaurants include soup or salad with dinner. Yes, it's going to take a lot of chattering and demonstration to convert the entire population from the mere acceptance of haircolor to the actual use of haircolor, but it seems to be destiny.

Haircolor Delivers Genuine Value and Benefits

When it comes to beauty and fashion, some have promised more than they could deliver. There have been all sorts of creams and potions and treatments that had a great story but provided little in the way of actual results. That's why governments stepped in years ago and prevented product manufacturers from making unsubstantiated claims.

The reality of haircolor is unmistakable! Haircolor is for real; it really does something. First, there is an actual external transformation that is predictable and lends itself to art. Haircolor obviously alters appearance and image. The effect of haircolor on how a person looks can be dramatic—a lingering effect that lasts not just an afternoon, but for weeks or months.

Second, with haircolor there is not only external transformation, but there is also an internal transformation that occurs. Haircolor effects people emotionally and psychologically. It has the power to alter how people feel about themselves, and this is its real power.

The psychological potency of haircolor gets to the heart of what consumers really want with image services. Dissatisfied with themselves before visiting the salon, people want to feel better when they leave. Haircolor delivers. After a haircolor service has been performed, people do feel differently about themselves. Haircoloring can help people feel better about themselves.

"Haircolor delivers both physical and mental transformation that impacts self-image as well as the first-impression judgment of others."

Haircolor makes people feel:

- *Younger*
- *Sexier*
- *Glamorous*
- *Desirable*
- *Popular*

- *Lovable*
- *Prestigious*
- *Fashionable*
- *Powerful*
- *Thin*

Haircolor has the power to profoundly impact a person's entire experience of life. Haircolor impacts self-image, self-esteem, self-confidence, and personal effectiveness.

If you have any doubt about how dramatic the psychological impact of haircolor is, consider for a moment the response when the guest is unhappy with the results. Tears flow—a pretty dramatic psychological response by anyone's measure. Fortunately, the overwhelming percentage of people only cry tears of joy!

Consider the profound positive psychological service performed with haircolor. That is one of the reasons why people with high aspirations about feeling good about themselves are such a natural market for haircolor. Haircolor delivers on its promises.

Third, not only does haircolor improve people's relationship with themselves, it also improves their relationships with others. It impacts on how people feel about themselves when interacting with others. Furthermore, it impacts how others will perceive and interact with them.

People respond to images, and color creates an unmistakable image. It is commonplace that people size up other people in a matter of seconds. People's hairstyle and haircolor are points of immediate observation. Color enables people to package themselves to get the response from others that they want. Whether it be the executive businesswoman or the country club socialite, the color of their hair can enhance people's ability to pull off the role they play and create the response they want to evoke from others.

Haircolor packs a powerful punch! When something not only affects a person externally, not only affects a person's internal psychological state, but also affects the image and status judgment of onlookers, that is something very powerful and very real to bring to the marketplace!

Everyone Has Access to Haircolor's Mystique

It's important to note that the entire population benefits from coloring, not just the baby boomers.

The youth population enjoys haircoloring as a coming of age ritual. This has gone on for years. It's a way for youth to express their individuality and personhood and to celebrate the youth culture and music. It's an opportunity to make an adult decision about who they are, the image they want to present to the world, and the tribe they want to run with.

True, a lot of these color applications are done at home. That's fine because as their spending power increases, they will come to the salon for haircolor having already experienced the mystique. Plus, haircolor is a healthy and more culturally vibrant way for young adults to assert their selfhood when contrasted with other possibilities such as taking up smoking, abusing alcohol, or experimenting with drugs.

Men color their hair. Millions of them do it. Almost all of them do it at home. Men color their hair for the very same reasons as women. Haircolor helps men feel better about how they look, and it improves the image they communicate to others.

The question is Why do so few men have their hair colored in the salon? Why do most opt to do it at home? Currently, only about 5 percent of male haircolor applications are performed in the salon. As we discuss in some detail later, a more focused and male-friendly packaging and presentation of color services can capture a much larger percentage of the male market. The point to understand now is that more men are sold on the practice of coloring their hair than the industry may realize.

> **"Salons can capture a much larger percentage of the male haircolor market through a more focused and male-friendly packaging and presentation of color services."**

The final point to make here is that many people feel that gray hair is unnecessary. Gray or graying hair can look simply dreadful on some middle-aged women. Some believe that gray hair is unflattering—a symbol of frumpyness and perhaps even laziness.

Many people can recall when cigarette smoking was thought to be suave and sophisticated. Now it is considered unhealthy and low class. So too with middle-aged gray hair. The implications of this are that others may judge middle-aged gray-haired folk as being undisciplined, unsophisticated, and perhaps out of fashion.

And it's all so unnecessary. We can rescue the gray haired from being outcast by insensitive and unthinking others and from beating themselves up needlessly about their appearance. Haircolor to the rescue!

There comes a time when we simply cross the line into the golden years and allow ourselves to be, act, and look older. Even then, color can improve senior hair by making it more ravishing, more full-bodied, and more stunning. So no one need ever graduate from the benefits of haircolor!

Haircolor Is Prestigious

Haircolor can offer prestige both to the salon as well as to the client. In fact, today nothing else in the salon offers the promise of prestige and exclusivity like haircolor.

Salons and designers who specialize in haircoloring enjoy a certain cachet. They distinguish themselves as possessing a level of artistry and sophistication beyond the ordinary. There is a special romance and magic surrounding haircolor, which is why haircolor specialists are held with such affection by their discriminating clientele. To be sure, haircoloring is an art. Any stylist can slap on some haircolor with fairly dependable results. But the master colorist who can deliver a superior design is today's role model in the industry.

This is one of the reasons why expert colorists command premium dollars and are the highest paid practitioners in the salon profession. In fact, the master colorist delights in a level of public respect and recognition equal to that of any professional. This is partly due to the extraordinarily high incomes they can command. And higher income for colorists means that the Age of Haircolor creates an environment allowing the profession to attract a higher caliber of individual to the ranks. Higher financial rewards have a tendency to do that.

Haircolor is also a prestige service for the consumer. First, it's a pampering service, so it has a luxury benefit. But more important, someone who wears quality haircolor is perceived as more wealthy, sophisticated, educated, successful, prosperous, comfortable, affluent, healthy, and desirable as a person. Today, haircolor is part of dressing for success. Masterfully executed, haircoloring can give someone the image of being well bred and of good stock. Haircolor can transform a lady from looking plain to looking like a million dollars!

Let it be said that this is not necessarily the image everyone aspires to. But also let it be said that haircolor can play a vital role in creating exactly the image each individual does aspire to. No matter what a client wants as an image, haircolor can deliver.

As more and more people wear quality professional color, the public will grow more and more sophisticated as to what good hair-coloring looks like. This is a process of consciousness raising.

The salon industry experienced the same thing with haircutting. It wasn't that many decades ago when the kitchen table dominated as the venue for haircuts. With the dawn of master cutters and wash-and-wear looks, salons were able to offer a dramatic comparative differ-ence. Soon enough ordinary folks were able to see the difference. Getting the haircut around the kitchen table simply did not deliver the goods. Because people have a tendency to be very self-critical when it comes to their appearance, walking around with an amateur haircut was too painful psychologically. The natural human need to feel and appear acceptable has meant that kitchen table haircuts have been in deep decline.

The same phenomenon is beginning to unfold with haircoloring. Home results simply will not be good enough anymore. The difference in results will be too dramatic when compared with what can be accomplished artistically in the salon. Consumers' self-consciousness and negative self-talk regarding the inadequacy of home coloring will compel people to convert to professional haircoloring by the millions (of patrons and dollars).

The desire for recognition and prestige, indeed the basic need to feel accepted and adequate, is incredibly strong. This is one of the reasons why professional haircolor market share will continue to grow dramatically. This also drives the industry's continuing efforts to refine its artistry and techniques. Professionals must package and present services so that they are most appealing to the consumer. It is time to more clearly distinguish professional haircoloring from home preparations.

Haircolor Promotes Loyalty through All Segments of the Business of Beauty

Like no other salon offering, haircolor is a loyalty service. When these patrons find a color department they like, they stick. Haircolor client retention can happen in much greater percentages that with cut and perm customers.

One reason for this is the mystery surrounding haircolor formulations and application techniques. The perception and reality are that a precise recipe must be followed to duplicate the look. The ability to create and consistently deliver a uniquely individual image is highly valued. So the loyalty of client to color department can be fanatical.

A second reason is that salons rarely change haircolor brands. Salons tend to give longer-term loyalty to color manufacturers than to perm or wet line brands. And because of the educational component associated with haircolor, distribution channels may be more stable. Consequently, there is a lot more willingness on the part of suppliers to genuinely help with technical and business ideas because there is a greater likelihood of a meaningful payback. With haircolor, everybody wins—which is fantastic for the industry. Haircolor encourages harmonious interaction and transaction.

Haircolor Maximizes Salon Income as well as Individual Opportunity

More income is good news. First, haircolor maximizes dollars received for time expended. It is a very time-efficient salon service for the money. The few minutes that it requires to design, formulate, apply, and rinse haircolor probably represents the highest pay for time designers enjoy. Plus, equipment and techniques that cut processing time can make matters even better.

Second, haircolor maximizes dollars per client visit. Because such a massive percentage of salon guests are realistic prospects for wearing haircolor and needing home maintenance products to keep it looking fresh, a real opportunity presents itself to increase guest spending dramatically. The fact that haircolor can be an impulse purchase only adds to the formula for big money. Numerous ways exist to entice practically all your visitors into haircolor. This reality will enable you to significantly increase the average value of each salon ticket.

> Haircolor creates stronger loyalty at all professional levels.

Third, haircolor has the subtle appeal that allows the professional to lead clients through progressively more sophisticated and expensive haircoloring services. A client introduced with a $20 application can be upgraded over time to a $100 service—something that cannot be done with a haircut!

Finally, haircolor lends itself to the team approach of client service, which is a real plus. Here's the way the big dollars are made. Imagine one master colorist with the assistance of two or three associates. The master colorist can take responsibility for consulting, designing, and overseeing the work of the design team. Each of the associates can be involved in client preparation, color mixing, application, overseeing proper processing, rinsing, conditioning, as well as some cutting and blow drying—depending on how the team functions.

Consider what this can accomplish financially. A colorist schedules four clients an hour—one at the top of the hour, one at ten after, another at twenty after, and the last one at half past. She has three associates who are paid $10 an hour—which, by the way, will attract high-quality practitioners in many metropolitan areas. After the master colorist consults with the client and designs the look, including haircolor, she turns the guest over to an associate. She then moves on to the next consultation. During her open 20 minutes at the end of each hour, she is able to spend additional individual time with each guest, providing the finishing touches to their style.

Imagine for the sake of example that her average ticket for color, cut, and style is $50—that is a conservative figure. Four clients at $50 each yields $200 an hour in revenues. Now she has to pay her help; so three associates at $10 each means $30 an hour labor expense. Deduct the $30 from the $200, and there is $170 to prorate between the designer and the shop. This is how the money is made. Everybody wins—from the consumer to the associates to the designer to the owner.

> The master colorist enjoys a level of respect, recognition, and income equal to that of any professional.

Granted, a team like this is not put together in a day. But it can be done. The scenario just described is a worthwhile aspiration for any salon professional. Time management and client flow must obviously be well choreographed to make this happen. Successful doctors' or dentists' offices offer a good model to emulate. Lower-level associates take care of all preliminary work. When the doctor or dentist comes in, he or she gets down to serious work at hand. When the doctor or dentist is finished, an associate returns to the room for any cleanup details. This is time management. Applications to the hair salon are obvious; financial enhancement is dramatic.

CONCLUSION

We are in the Age of Haircolor. Haircolor provides the greatest opportunity that this industry will enjoy this generation!

> **"Opportunity for high income has never been greater!"**

If there was ever a time when a cosmetologist could enjoy high aspirations and great possibilities, this is it! Welcome to real prosperity in the Age of Haircolor!

In this chapter, we discovered the following:

1. *Haircolor delivers customers. The public has demonstrated that they want, and will pay for, haircoloring.*
2. *Haircolor delivers style. It has now become an essential component of fashion and is evolving to the point where it is a universal cultural phenomenon.*
3. *Haircolor delivers genuine external and internal benefits that are highly desirable.*
4. *Haircolor delivers benefits for the entire population in a healthy and uplifting style.*
5. *Haircolor delivers a level of approval, recognition, and prestige to both the public and the practitioner. Everybody who touches haircolor can be transformed by its charms.*
6. *Haircolor delivers loyalty. Consumers and practitioners know enough not to mess around with formulas that work.*
7. *People who deliver so much powerful and transformational value to the marketplace attract money. Haircolor increases the flow of currency. One of the laws of money is that money automatically flows to value. The more value you create and deliver to others, the more the forces of abundance and prosperity are set into motion. Appreciate the transformational power of haircolor.*

Part One:
Planning to Build Your
Haircolor Business

"Plan your work and work your plan." When Dale Carnegie coined that expression, he hit upon the truth of progress. Determine your goals and then make a plan to accomplish them. Establish milestones to gauge your progress. Then go full out to implement your plan of action.

To grow your haircolor income, you must first be absolutely convinced of the value of consistent effort. Progress comes by relentlessly introducing professional haircoloring to all your salon guests. Second, you must make a commitment to set specific and measurable goals and to track your progress faithfully.

The primary purpose in this section is to reveal specifically what you need to do to see your haircolor income go up. You will know the goals to set and how to calculate your progress.

In "Planning to Build Your Haircolor Business," you discover
1. how haircolor can dramatically boost your income.
2. why you must establish clear goals.
3. the five golden formulas for million-dollar haircolor marketing.
  a. How to calculate haircolor market penetration
  b. How to calculate haircolor income share
  c. How to calculate your average service ticket
  d. How to calculate color services per guest
  e. How to build $100 tickets

How Haircolor Can Dramatically Boost Your Income

First, convince yourself that haircolor can significantly alter the quality of your financial life as a professional designer. If you have not already discovered it, you will soon learn that salon guests will purchase haircolor on impulse. Imagine for a moment what would happen if just one extra visitor a day elected to have his or her hair colored.

> Make a commitment to set specific, measurable goals and to track your progress faithfully.

Colors and highlights are priced all over the spectrum, so for simplicity imagine that the average haircolor service yielded a $50 purchase. Also, imagine that you work at the salon 250 days per year. Look what happens to your income with one extra color client a day:

$$\$50 \times 250 \text{ days} = \$12,500!$$

Not too shabby! Each salon has its own pay program, but any designer would end up with thousands and thousands of dollars worth of extra income and benefits as a result of this extra activity.

Now start to look six months down the road when all these new color clients are coming back regularly for touch-ups and freshening of their colors. Not only do you service them, but each new day you continue to generate one new impulse purchase of coloring. It's as if you are now doing two extra colors per day. Compare this to where you started from. Instead of generating extra income at the rate of $12,500 per year, in six months, you are generating extra income at the rate of $25,000 per year.

Are you ready to start shopping for that new car yet? And then imagine what happens one year, eighteen months, or two years down the road! And this is not multilevel marketing! This is the reality of haircolor income.

Look to the day when demand for your services grows beyond the point of the amount of haircolor applications you can personally supply. With haircolor, you can start to leverage yourself through the assistance of an associate. Now you can do nearly twice as many patrons. And the laws of economics teach us that with higher demand you can increase your prices because you are in limited supply. Have you started to get a feel for how your income can grow with haircolor?

This all happens with your commitment to stimulate just one impulse purchase of haircolor per day. For some, these numbers may seem astonishing, but they are the reality of what happens when you consistently and enthusiastically promote color to each and every salon guest whom you encounter. A personal example will help you see the bigger picture.

> **"Enticing one additional salon guest into the haircolor arena today creates instant bonus income and sets the stage for compounded bonus income tomorrow."**

I know of a young man who has been out of cosmetology school less than five years and who follows the principles I share throughout this program. On a good day at the salon, with one associate helping him, he does over $1,000 in business. This is not just the day before Christmas. He will achieve this a number of times each month. In fact, on a really good day he hits the $1,500 mark.

This is not some Madison Avenue hot-shot here. This is a salt of the earth, hard working professional named Jerry who works in a country salon outside of Atlanta, Georgia. And, he is not unique. There are a number of associates at that same salon who rack up comparable numbers!

My experience owning and operating salons means I know that these kinds of results are not common. Most stylists are tickled if they can do $300 a day; $500 a day is beyond the imagination of the vast majority of hairstylists now working in North America. But in communities large and small, all around the continent, the $1,000 mark can be achieved—as a matter of fact, it is being achieved.

Even if you get only halfway there, that's $500 in services a day. For most a $500 daily take would represent a very dramatic impact both in terms of financial status and quality of life.

Stimulating impulse purchasing of haircolor is definitely worth your time as a designer. And if you are an owner or manager, study the numbers and you can immediately see why now is the Age of Haircolor.

Why You Must Establish Clear Goals

Where are you right now? It sounds simple, but to get to where you want to go, you first have to know where you are. This requires a little bit of number crunching. One of the rules of goal setting is to establish goals that can be quantified and measured.

Paying attention to specific and measurable goals can automatically effect how you see each interaction with a guest. If you have specific and measurable goals, then how you behave, what you say, and the direction that your salon conversations take are all affected. That's one of the reasons why setting and reviewing goals makes professionals far more effective and far more focused on accomplishment.

"Specific, written, measureable goals that are reviewed regularly give direction, motivation, and focus to your haircolor income growth plans."

For example, early in the Age of Retail, yet not that long ago, many salons had a single facing of a few products on display in a glass case under lock and key. At some point the industry began to establish criteria about what good retail performance meant from an objective, numerical standpoint.

Have you ever heard that salons should aspire to a retail percentage equal to 25 percent of service sales? Back in 1970 most salons were doing one tenth of 25 percent. But once salons started measuring retail performance, the increase in performance began to show itself at once. People got creative, thinking of new ways to introduce and demonstrate products. People began to merchandise and display more effectively. As business grew, some major manufacturers began to support salon industry efforts with outstanding ad campaigns in consumer magazines and on television. In a matter of years, retail sales at salons increased tenfold. That's what can happen when you focus your efforts and have specific and measurable goals.

Exactly the same thing will happen with haircolor during the generation ahead. More and more of the population will experience the ongoing benefits of haircoloring, and an increasingly larger percentage of them will opt for salon coloring services over home coloring.

The Five Golden Formulas for Million-Dollar Haircolor Marketing

Five easy and specific calculations help measure and motivate improved performance. They are affectionately called "The Five Golden Formulas for Million-Dollar Haircolor Marketing."

#1. How to Calculate Haircolor Market Penetration

Whether you are a salon owner or a hair designer, your clientele is your current market. How much of that market have you penetrated with professional haircoloring? Specifically, what percentage of your salon guests use your haircoloring services?

Haircolor market penetration is easy to calculate. Simply divide the number of guests with haircolor by the total number of guests to determine your haircolor market penetration.

> **Guests having haircoloring ÷ Total guests =**
> **Haircolor market penetration**

For example, last week, of your 40 salon guests, 5 had their hair colored. Your market penetration is 5/40 = .125, or 12½ percent.

Yesterday, of 10 guests, only 1 had haircoloring. Your market penetration is 1/10 = .1, or 10 percent.

To start, find out where you are right now. Go over your personal records and count back the last 100 guests. How many of them had haircolor during their visit? If it was 6, then your market penetration was 6 percent. If it was 14, then your penetration was 14 percent. If it was 28, then your penetration was 28 percent.

Whatever your current market penetration, consider it okay. It is okay to be wherever you are. Wherever you are, plant your feet firmly so that you can step ahead and proceed.

Before discussing some ideas on how to set your goals for market penetration growth, let's review some vital statistics. It appears that in 1996, apparently 18 percent of salon visitors in the United States purchased coloring services at salons. If your clientele is predominantly male, your numbers are apt to be softer. If your clientele is predominantly female, your numbers could be firmer. Those are the averages.

> *Rule of Thumb:*
> * *For a typical salon, 33 percent haircolor market penetration*
> * *For a color specialty salon, 90 percent haircolor market penetration*

What can your haircolor market penetration grow to? What can you aspire to? Imagine having one in three guests buying haircolor. As a rule of thumb for an average salon, a minimum of one third of guests should purchase a haircolor service. But then, how about one in two? Or how about two out of three? Wouldn't that be something? Go for three out of four?

Imagine the impact on your quality of life if three out of four visitors purchased haircoloring services from you each day. What would this do to your financial picture? What kind of an impact would it have on the home you live in, the furnishings you enjoy, your wardrobe, where you eat, the schools your children attend, the car you drive, the vacations you experience, the feelings of peace and ease and security you enjoy? In reality, consider the impact on the stability and security of your financial life and all the opportunity and peace of mind that go with a 75 percent haircolor market penetration. If all you had to do was get three out of four guests involved in haircoloring, wouldn't it be worth it?

How about increasing those numbers to four out of five, or five out of six, or six out of seven, or seven out of eight, or eight out of nine, or maybe even nine out of ten? Imagine, nine out of ten visitors with professional haircolor!

A salon owner in Marietta, Georgia, calculated that between 92 percent and 93 percent of their salon guests purchase haircoloring. If you saw how their operation functions, you would realize that a lot of their first time visitors have no idea they are going to be purchasing haircolor when they first walk through the door. They buy haircolor on impulse. Soon you will learn about the ways the salon team achieves this.

For now, start right where you are with the market penetration you calculated for yourself and set some goals for the future. Following are some ideas that will help.

DAILY GOALS

How about setting specific goals for each day? Much can happen very quickly with focused effort. The designer who usually performs color services on one out of ten guests can get to four or five out of ten in a matter of days. That can happen when you direct your energy and enthusiasm and utilize the resources already at hand. Do not make a six month project out of something that can happen in six days. The beauty of haircolor is that you can start right now right from where you are. The only thing that can possibly hold you back is your own fear— of failure, of rejection, of inadequacy. Without going into a lot of detail, you must govern yourself by the sunshine of opportunity and faith and avoid turning your eyes to the darkness of fear.

> **"Salon professionals can experience dramatic growth in haircolor market penetration overnight with focused effort and desire."**

MID-RANGE GOALS

Set longer-term goals—like one week, one month, and three months. You want to set longer-term goals to make sure that your effort is consistent. It is not enough to do beaucoup color services for a couple of days and then leave it alone. Getting the job done day in and day out over a prolonged period of time makes the fortune. It is pointless to start fast only to fizzle out. Get a fast start and maintain a consistent pace so that you can win the marathon. The more practice you have giving haircolor consultations, the more effective you will become and the greater the percentage of patrons who will take you up on your proposal.

BE PASSIONATE ABOUT FOLLOWING YOUR PROGRESS

Every day, every week, every month make it your first priority to count your totals to see how you are progressing. Celebrate your market share growth. Constantly think about what you can do or say to improve your performance. Eat, breathe, drink, walk haircolor and you will make great strides very quickly.

#2. How to Calculate Haircolor Income Share

Market penetration tells us the percentage of guests buying professional haircolor. Income share tells us the percentage of salon service revenues that flow from haircolor. What percentage of your service revenues are coming from haircolor?

Haircolor income share is easy to calculate. But before that, let's make one important distinction. When you have service packages that include haircolor, you need to determine the value of the haircolor itself to make this calculation valid. Say you do a color and cut for $58. How much of that $58 is for color and how much is for the cut? You need to prorate it so that you can look at the haircolor revenue independently and get a pure read on your haircolor income share.

Here's the equation. To determine your haircolor income share, divide your total haircolor income by your total service income.

**Total haircolor income ÷ Total service income =
Haircolor income share**

For example, last week you generated $230 in haircolor sales out of $920 in total service sales.

$$\$230 \div \$920 = .25$$

So your haircolor income share was 25 percent of total service income.

Or perhaps yesterday you did $40 in haircolor sales out of $200 total service sales. Then $40/$200 = .2, or 20 percent of your revenues came from haircolor.

As in determining your market penetration, you start this by finding out where you are right now. Go over your personal records and calculate your total service sales (not including retail) over the last 30 days. How many dollars worth of haircolor services did you sell in that time? What percentage of your total service sales were your haircolor sales?

Right now do not make any judgments; just see where you are starting from. The number can be high or low. The issue is where will it be tomorrow? You need to have something to measure against as you start to work with the concepts in this program.

Before setting your personal goals, consider the following data. A recent survey found that haircolor sales make up about 23 percent of salon service income. Those numbers may be a bit high. The largest chains yield less than 20 percent of service sales from haircolor. One of the most respected department store chains has haircolor income share in the 17 to 18 percent range. Further, most of the mass market chains that focus on cutting services typically generate less than 5 percent of their service income from color sales.

Today, the strongest haircolor sales are coming from independent salons. An income share of 35 percent to 40 percent is not uncommon among top salons that emphasize color. A few salons are able to generate 50 percent or more of their service revenues from the haircolor service.

Granted, there are some exclusive "color only" salons that generate practically all of their dollars from haircolor. But there are probably less than 50 of these businesses among the more than 150,000 salons operating in North America. The numbers being discussed here relate more to salons that offer an array of services to guests.

Now, keeping in mind the thoughts about setting daily goals, about establishing longer-term goals, and being passionate about your advancement and progress, begin the practice of planning specific and measurable goals for haircolor income share growth.

Know definitively what you want to accomplish and get it down on paper. Where do you want your haircolor income share to be today? this week? this month? in 60 or 90 days? Get it down on paper. Write it in the first person, present tense. Be very specific: "On December 15, 25 percent of my service income flows from haircolor sales." "On January 15, 30 percent of my service income flows from haircolor sales." "On February 15, 35 percent of my service income flows from haircolor sales." Hang your written goals on the wall in the dispensary; tape them to your bathroom mirror; put them on your windshield. Be passionate about it!

#3. How to Calculate Your Average Service Ticket

Start to calculate the average value of your service tickets. Your tickets probably include everything from bang trims to corrective coloring. But, what is the average? You will discover that the more haircolor you do on more guests, the higher your average ticket.

It is easy to calculate your average salon ticket. You simply take your total service dollars (before taxes—and don't count retail purchases!) and divide by the number of customers you served.

> **Total service dollars ÷ Number of customers =**
> **Average service ticket**

Take a look at the total spent for services by your last 100 customers. Say it was $2,000. Divide by 100, and your average service ticket was $20.

Say that your last 100 guests spent $1,825 on services. Again, divide $1,825 by 100, and $18.25 was your average service ticket.

What is your average service ticket? Remember this rule of thumb: *Your average service ticket should be at least twice the price of your haircut.* That's important, so repeat it again and again to yourself for emphasis.

Say that your haircut is priced at $15. Your average service ticket should be $30 or more. So often in my consultation practice I find salons with a haircut price of $20 and an average ticket of $23.64 or $22.31. That simply is not good enough! If you are in this range, then you are simply not stimulating enough impulse service purchases of treatments or haircolor.

> *Rule of Thumb:*
> *Your average service ticket should be at least twice the price of your haircut!*

Once again, calculate where you are right now and then set goals for immediate improvement. And once you get your average service ticket up to twice the value of a haircut, keep on going. Try to increase it to three times the price. Compete with yourself to advance your personal best.

#4. How to Calculate Color Services per Guest

If you haven't already, you'll quickly discover that you should endeavor to perform multiple color services on each client. First of all, because that is what real artistic design work requires, and second, because that is where the greatest spending occurs.

Recall that one of the real virtues of color is its appeal and there-fore its capability to evolve a client's spending on color services from $20 to over $100. This is largely accomplished by performing increas-ingly more elaborate and complicated color work. Performing multiple services during each visit is the path to higher income.

For example, the colorist prepares the canvas with a semiperma-nent color, then adds dimensional highlights, then performs a glossing service to maximize shine and luster. Finally, the colorist touches up the eyebrows to create a cohesive and dramatic look. That's four services, and it could go further!

Once market penetration is happening, the next major effort is to continually introduce color clients to increasingly sophisticated and elaborate procedures. When looking for measurable progress, you must have an objective measure that you can count. The number of color services per client provides that.

You can start your own analysis, historically, by reviewing the last 100 clients you saw and counting not only which ones had color, but how many color services each had. Many will have had just one. A few may have had two. Did any have three on a given visit? Or four? Add them all up and divide by the 100 guests and see how many color services you performed per salon guest. Here's the simple equation:

**Total number of color services ÷ Number of guests =
Color services per guest**

If you performed a total of 50 color services on your last 100 guests, then you performed .5 color services per guest, one half of a color service per guest.

If you had performed a total of 125 color services on your last 100 guests, then you would have performed 1.25 color services per guest. Your goal should be to get that "color services per guest" number over 1. That will be a sure sign that you are making progress. This is a good rule of thumb to shoot for: at least one color service per salon guest.

Another way to proceed is to look at the number of color services per color client. Because not every client wears color, how many color services are you able to perform, on average, on those who do wear color?

**Number of color services ÷ Number of color clients =
Color services per color client**

Simply divide the number of color services performed by the number of guests they were performed on to determine the number of color services per color client.

#5. How to Build $100 Tickets

How many $100 tickets are you writing? With haircolor you can get clients over the $100 mark—one of the real benefits of emphasizing haircolor. How many of us can get away with a $100 haircut or even a $50 haircut? What kind of a perm wrap and how much time would you have to spend to justify a $100 perm bill? You would probably be working on it all afternoon! With great time efficiency you can perform a multiservice haircolor makeover and achieve the $100 price point. For some higher-end salons it may be the $200 threshold you will want to break.

The $100 ticket is something to be approached with boldness. Sometimes stylists themselves have a tendency to shy away from this ticket level. I have personally witnessed a hairstylist rewrite a ticket that should have been $104 into one for $93. Then she put it on the front counter and made a bee line for the back before the customer had a chance to react to the price! She wanted to be out of the way of the customer's wrath when she saw the check! This is crazy!

Our own psychological hang-ups hold us back. I have tapes and programs that deal with "The Moment of Insanity." These deal with self-esteem, self-image, and self-talk issues. Fear-based thinking holds people back from achieving what they are capable of. We could spend hours talking about the internal demons that plague us all. Suffice it to say, your work is worth the $100 ticket.

The transformation and happiness you can bring to your clients have the power to impact their day-to-day experience of life. Their self-esteem, their self-confidence, their feeling good about themselves, their interactions with other people are all influenced by your color work. Put full energy into the contribution you make. Recognize its value.

Do not short change your customers. Do not give them less than what you are capable of because of your own fear-based hang-ups. Give them all that you can and realize that we live in a universe of boundless abundance. There is a prize to enjoy. Do not relegate yourself and your clients to some second-class, less-than-the-best offering simply because of your own hang-ups about money.

Remember the old rhyme:

I bargained with life for a penny and life would pay no more.
No matter how I begged in the evening when I counted my
scanty store. For life is just an employer. It gives you what you
ask. And, once you have set the wages, you must bear the
task. I know. I once worked for a menials hire. Only to learn
dismayed, that any wage I have asked of life, life would
willingly pay.

Face your fears. Focus on abundance rather than lack. Let the
sunshine light your path, and do not set your sights on impoverished
thinking about limitations and lack. You get out of life what you expect.
Check your thinking. You are in control of the messages you give yourself. If you constantly think, "I'm not going to have enough money to pay
my bills" and "my clients can't afford any more than what they're paying
right now," then you are sending very specific messages to yourself.

Current psychological thinking teaches that your goal-seeking,
automatic-pilot subconscious computer does not judge the merit or
truth of the messages you give it. It just acts about your programming.
And, as any computer programmer can testify, "junk in, junk out."

Consider the consequences. If you think, "I'm not going to have
enough money to pay my bills," then your subconscious mind will see
to it that you do not have enough money to pay your bills. You asked
for it! That was the instruction you gave. If you dictate, "My clients can't
afford any more than what they're paying right now," then those are
the clients you are going to get and that will be your reality. This thinking is not new. Saints and sages from earliest days shared this truth.

Partnered with impoverished thinking is the problem of scarcity
thinking. It goes like this: Many people have been accustomed to making so little money that $100 sounds like a lot of money. It isn't any-
more. In this day and age, $100 is not that much money. Not many of
us were raised in a family that had a lot of extra money to throw
around, and so we are not used to spending $100 on ourselves.
Therefore we think that others also will find this amount excessive.

These days, people spend $100 at a restaurant for a dinner that is
forgotten by morning. You would probably be surprised how many of

your customers spend that much at the department store for cosmetics and skin care and think nothing of it.

> You receive what you believe. Those who deeply believe that their clients would not spend $100 will surely receive clients who will not spend $100.

Once you are psychologically prepared to approach and break the $100 barrier with boldness, here's what you do. Go back over the last month and see how many guests spent over $100 or $200, as the case may be, on services. How does that come out in total numbers? How does that come out as a percentage of total guests?

Say that in the last month you had 100 guests and that 6 of them exceeded $100 in service purchases. That is 6 percent of your guests spending over $100 on services.

You know what to do next: Start looking at each and every guest as someone for whom you can make a difference, a $100 difference. Set your goals for today and for this week. How many $100 service tickets are you going to write? Decide this in advance. Plan the results you want, then do what it takes. Deliver the service level you must deliver to get there. Now set 30-, 60-, and 90-day goals to dramatically improve the percentage of guests spending over $100 with color as your strategy. I know you can do it—and so do you.

A final point to think about is that once you get people over the $100 psychological threshold, it is relatively easy to keep them spending more on that visit. So do not stop at $100. The next major psychological barrier does not really come until the $200 mark, so continue to $150 and then to $190 by adding additional color services and retail items. Add on increasingly as the client is in the makeover mood!

Use Table 2-1 to calculate
a. your haircolor market penetration.
b. your haircolor income share.
c. your average service ticket.
d. your color services per guest.
e. your $100 tickets.

Table 2-1   Haircolor Success Formula Status Sheet

		FORMULA		Starting Point	Week 1	Week 2	Week 3	Week 4
Service Guests	#1	Count #	Goal					
			Actual					
			Over/Under					
Service Income	#2	Count $	Goal					
			Actual					
			Over/Under					
Average Service Ticket	#3	#2 / #1 = #3 Answer is $	Goal					
			Actual					
			Over/Under					
Haircolor Guests	#4	Count #	Goal					
			Actual					
			Over/Under					
Haircolor Market Penetration	#5	#4 / #1 = #5 Answer is %	Goal					
			Actual					
			Over/Under					
Haircolor Income	#6	Count $	Goal					
			Actual					
			Over/Under					
Haircolor Income Share	#7	#6 / #2 = #7 Answer is %	Goal					
			Actual					
			Over/Under					
Color Services	#8	Count #	Goal					
			Actual					
			Over/Under					
Color Services per Guest	#9	#8 / #1 = #9 Answer is #	Goal					
			Actual					
			Over/Under					
Color Services per Color Guest	#10	#8 / #4 = #10 Answer is #	Goal					
			Actual					
			Over/Under					
$100.00 Service Tickets	#11	Count # Answer is #	Goal					
			Actual					
			Over/Under					

Part Two:
Positioning Yourself and
Your Salon for Haircolor

Salons and designers who situate themselves as haircolor specialists will be in a position to make more money than other cosmetologists.

In "Positioning Yourself and Your Salon for Haircolor" you learn
1. why specialists tend to make more money.
2. how specialization actually expands opportunity.
3. two alternative ways to specialize with haircolor.
4. principles of color department layout.

Why Specialists Tend to Make More Money

A common mistake that salons make is that they try to be everything
for everybody. Fearful that asserting a specialty could run off some
clients, most salons opt for the image of the generalist. The general
salon practitioner, jack of all trades and services, is how most cosmetologists position themselves.

In any field of endeavor—whether it be the doctor, lawyer,
accountant, carpenter, butcher, baker, or candlestick maker—generalists
tend to make considerably less than specialists. The brain surgeon
enjoys more income and status than the family practitioner. In the age

> **"An expert is a person who has made all the mistakes which can be made in a very narrow field."**
>
> —Neils Bohr

of specialization, the specialist reigns supreme.

There are two primary reasons why specialists make more money. First, they know more. They become extremely well versed in their specialty. Consider the truth of that statement by the famous scientist Neils Bohr. Second, people will pay a premium for the extra measure of confidence and quality they expect from someone with extensive specialized experience.

How Specialization Actually Expands Opportunity

One of the real benefits of haircolor is that it enables you to enhance the amount of money you can make per unit of time. The more haircolor you do, the fewer other less-lucrative services you have time to perform. The value of your time is enriched. That is the opportunity of specialization.

In the salon profession, many people avoid specialization because of fear they could be limiting their market. Consider this dose of reality. You have a limited supply of yourself to sell anyway. There are only so many hours in a day, and you have only two hands. The realities of time and space automatically limit the number of people you can personally serve.

Even if you are in a small community, it is not necessary for you to be all things to all people. Consider the following example. If you do 12 customers a day, five days a week, and they return every six weeks, then you have a total of 12 x 5 x 6 customers, or 360 salon clients. That's it. That's how many you can effectively handle. You do not need any more than that. If only a few thousand people live in your market area, then you have all the opportunity that you need. If each client averages just $300 a year in services with you, which is very achievable as a color specialist, then multiply 360 clients by $300 and you have $108,000 in service tickets annually. Add retail and tips and as an employee you would be making well over $50,000 a year.

If you are really ambitious, you can have a couple of associates enhancing your productivity to where you can process 30 clients a day. Even then you are able to handle, at best, only a thousand total clients. You do not need, you cannot handle, and you do not want to have everybody as a customer. You want the customers who are willing to spend premium dollars for your specialization. That is where the money is.

You have heard others say that you can and should choose the clientele you want. That is exactly what specialization is all about. With haircolor, instead of merely choosing pleasant neighborhood residents, you focus on the pleasant residents who can and will pay for quality haircoloring services. That's the niche you choose, the market you develop. Make a decision to specialize and a marketing commitment to identify those who want your specialty.

Plus, specialization leaves plenty of room for general practice. You can specialize in haircolor without eliminating other service opportunities.

Think about restaurants that specialize, even the most basic hamburger chains like McDonald's. McDonald's is primarily identified as a hamburger establishment. However, you the patron know that you can get a chicken or fish sandwich, Mexican foods, a salad, pie and ice cream, pizza, eggs and pancakes, Danish, and a whole variety of beverages. So, even though their primary niche is hamburgers, they still can and do provide a whole array of foods that people want.

On the other side of the price spectrum, consider the most deluxe steak house in your town. You can probably order pork ribs, chicken, fish, shrimp, and lobster off the same menu with their specialty of steaks.

Even as you establish your clear identity with haircolor, you can still easily and freely offer the entire array of other salon services without any problem whatsoever. All the while, keep positioning for haircolor with all the benefits that specialization provides.

And it's not just haircolor. The industry is seeing the emergence of more and more full-service salons and spas.

> Proclaiming a haircolor specialty still leaves the door wide open to offer any additional salon services you wish.

Specializing in color services, including make-up and nail artistry, can provide a unique position in the marketplace. Day spas and full-service salons, which traditionally have gone the generalist route, can use color to distinguish themselves from the competition.

In "The Color Spa," an article in *DaySpa Magazine*, I wrote the following:

> *What does the public think of when they hear "day spa"? Images of facials, massage, body therapy and various other toning and skin treatments come to mind. Relaxation, rejuvenation, cleansing, health and hygiene. While luxury and pampering are part of the imagery, high fashion and glamour aren't necessarily part of the equation. In fact, hair and nail and make-up services are more associated with "full service salons" than with day spas.*
>
> *Typically at the day spa, after the pedicure, facial, waxing and massage the client is asked if they would like to have their hair washed and blown out before they hit the street. This is a very common situation. And, while the client may feel wonderful they often look horrible with dishevelled hair and blotchy skin when they emerge from a session of treatments. The finished has been overlooked.*
>
> *Color can be your "unique selling proposition". By simply adding color or emphasising it more you are able to bring a much more comprehensive offering into play. Talk about "full service" and color becomes essential. Color enables you to go full circle with the client and finish the look by packaging the appearance. Color is the accessory and the day spa that can coordinate the accessories and deliver them with style will situate itself uniquely and exclusively in any community. It's what can differentiate you from your competition.*

The point is that you can use color as your "unique selling proposition" without slowing demand for your other services one little bit. In fact it can only help matters and position you more exclusively and for a stronger market image and higher price points.

Two Alternative Ways to Specialize with Haircolor

Before we get into some of the specific techniques you can use for specialization, there are two roads you can travel. The first option is to position yourself essentially as a color practitioner and your business as a color emporium. The second strategy is to departmentalize and to create a specific color identity within your salon enterprise.

The Color Emporium

With "The Color Emporium," you clearly and unequivocally develop an image and situate your practice as being primarily one of color. The very name of your business says color in the mind of the consumer. You may even choose a name that shouts color. Here are some salon names you may find interesting.

The Artists Room	*Crayons*
Beaux Arts	*Golden Images*
A Blaze of Color	*Hot Reds*
Blondies	*Hues*
The Color Emporium	*Kaleidoscope*
The Color Room	*MagiColors*
Colors	*Painted Lady*
The Color Spa	*Shades*

Let your imagination run wild!

If you already have an established name that is well known in the marketplace, you may not want to sacrifice that good will by changing your name. In such cases, you will find that the use of a slogan can position your specialty as a hair-color business.

A slogan is something than can be appended to your existing name. "Jonathan's—Your Place for Color Makeover Magic!" Or, "The Metropolitan Salon and Spa—Your Color Authority."

"You can use a slogan to identify your hair-color specialty without losing the good will of the salon name you have established in the marketplace."

Once you decide on a slogan, include it every time your business name appears. In fact, have your slogan graphically included as a part of your logo.

The Color Department

The second positioning strategy is to have a clearly differentiated color department within your salon. Before we discuss the physical layout and reality of the color department, let's address the color department from the perspective of market identity.

Ideally, you want to imbue your color department with its own particular image in the marketplace. That is where your greatest positioning power is. For example, we have all heard of Mr. Goodwrench as a place for car repairs. We can visualize the image that Mr. Goodwrench has created in the marketplace. He has his own logo, his own uniform, his own slogans, his own personality and identity.

> For added distinction in the marketplace, consider positioning your color department as if it were a unique entity.

Now where do you find Mr. Goodwrench? Mr. Goodwrench has done such a good job of creating his own identity that most people have forgotten that he is really the General Motors Service Department at your local GM dealer. That is departmentalization done with excellence and clarity—no confusion here, no mixed messages. It has been done so well that most people do not even link Mr. Goodwrench with GM. When they think Mr. Goodwrench, they simply think auto service and auto repair.

That level of differentiation should convey your specialty with color. So, occupying the premises with The Town and Country Salon and Spa is The Magic Color Room, which occupies a distinct area of the salon strictly devoted to color services. The Magic Color Room would have its own logo, its own promotional campaign, its own signage, its own staff and uniform, its own identity in the marketplace.

Also, when you think departmentalization, think synergy. The coffee shop in the bookstore is an example of synergy. The two play off one another. Starbucks helps Barnes and Noble attract shoppers who linger longer. There is a correlation between length of visit and amount purchased from a retail store. Barnes and Noble helps Starbucks build traffic and provides people a reason to linger and enjoy a coffee with a new or contemplated book purchase. These two work together beautifully!

> **"Departmentalization can yield synergies and cross-promotional opportunities not available to more typical salons."**

Naturally, The Town and Country Salon and Spa and The Magic Color Room have a synergy that you would want to exploit. Actually, by positioning them as two separate entities, you can play one off the other with more power than you would expect. You can create endless possibilities to cross-sell and cross-promote as you make a visit to your place of business more exciting for the consumer.

Some people who are exposed to this information understand the concept but do not relate it to their own business. If this is true of you, it may be due to the size of your existing location or that you are renting a station. Let me first assure you that you will continue to find countless strategies that will prove to be of immediate and practical use. But beyond that, challenge yourself—and your colleagues—to aspire to more. The title here could be *Million Dollar Haircolor Income* because you deserve to know what you have the option to pursue if you so desire.

The bottom line is that to maximize your haircolor income you need to establish and emphasize your identity as a salon specializing in haircoloring. Either of the two methods just described here enables you to create your image and reputation as the place for dependable and beautiful haircoloring in your community.

As we continue, you will learn a whole smorgasbord of techniques you can use to master either of the two positioning options just described or some hybrid you concoct. Before delving into those methods, we must address the important topic of salon layout as it relates to positioning for color.

Principles of Color Department Layout

The layout of your salon or color department is the easiest and most direct way to demonstrate and dramatize your standing as a hair-coloring specialist. Ideally you need to fashion three interrelated components:

- The application zone
- The consultation zone
- The formulation zone

These zones are separate, unique, distinct areas within the salon or spa that are devoted to color. The haircolor consultation, application, and formulation areas must be well defined from the cutting, styling, or comb-out stations. (See Figure 2-1.) This is a very important positioning move.

People will buy haircolor on impulse, but consultation must be effective. A haircolor department establishes the kind of automatic authority necessary to dissolve many client fears. Your color services will be the mainstay of your impulse purchase up-sell strategy. As such they must be situated in high-traffic, well-exposed areas of the salon or spa. The consultation and especially the application areas must be located in highly visible spots. Ideally, place them in the center of the main floor. This positioning allows for maximum showmanship and excitement around the service, which in turn maximizes appeal and impulse purchasing.

Showmanship is an important selling tool with color services. Use all the bells and whistles to make haircoloring services extra fun. Use color to give the client recognition as the center of attention. Make sure that your physical layout amplifies the value of the show-manship you bring into play. Anything that focuses attention on your color zones will reward you with additional color interest among salon patrons and help to stimulate impulse purchasing.

The Application Zone

Your haircolor application area needs to be right out in the middle of the salon floor. In the most successful salons, this is one of the reasons

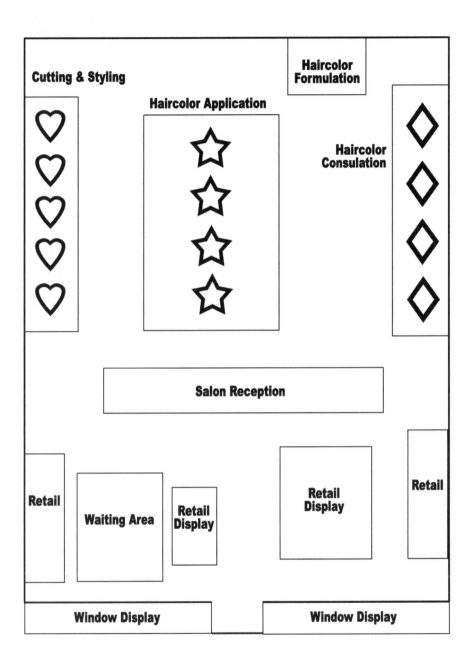

FIGURE 2-1. Salon layout illustrating consultation, application, and formulation zones

over 90 percent of the salon clients benefit from professional haircolor. What makes this fact even more remarkable is that many of those visitors do not even anticipate that they will be purchasing haircolor when they first arrive. They buy on impulse.

The color department layout captivates new guests. It attracts attention, creates interest, and builds haircolor desire among new salon patrons—so successfully in fact that virtually all guests will purchase haircolor services, many of them impulsively.

To hide haircolor application in a corner or behind a screen or even in a separate room is a major mistake. That approach takes the fun out of the process and makes it seem to everyone that haircolor is messy or ought to be kept a secret somehow. That is not the direction to go with this.

A word about male haircolor application. It remains a common misconception among salon professionals that men want some kind of exceptional privacy when their hair is being colored. That is nonsense. Some pretty remarkable salons have constructed special private areas for their male clientele only to discover that the men actually prefer to be out with everyone else. Today, men can generally handle being in a haircolor application zone. The young and early middle-age generations definitely can handle it. It behooves us as an industry to encourage men to be completely comfortable with all aspects of professional haircolor. Some people maintain that men want their own shops to go to, and they cite market research to back up this claim. I contend that none of the efforts along those lines has proven itself in the marketplace.

> Position the haircolor application zone in a high visability area. Use maximum showmanship when applying color to make the service fun and to give color clients recognition.

Also, the common practice of each designer applying haircolor at his or her cutting station is not ideal. It simply does not allow the kind of showmanship, recognition, or emphasis that is proven to work best. The added appeal of group participation really helps stimulate the impulse purchase of haircolor. That appeal is lost when everything is done at the cutting station.

Sometimes people in booth rental environments ask me how they can have a separate application area when they are confined to their station. My recommendation is for the entire salon to create a common area for color consultation and application that all designers can use. It's much like the common areas for reception, waiting, and retail that are typical of station rental environments. Naturally, devoting key areas of salon floor space to a haircolor common area requires that booth rental rates will need adjustment. However, the opportunity for added income is so dramatic that a rental adjustment is minuscule by comparison.

In fact, owners of booth rental salons should consider carefully some of the layout suggestions being made here. Creating a color friendly environment could be your unique selling proposition to top colorists in your area. Don't be just another booth rental salon. Have a special niche of the market that sets you apart.

To distinguish the application zone, you can use suspended signage, special flooring, an elevated island, unique lighting, canopies, awnings, and similar architectural devices.

You can certainly start off simply with rubber floor mats, differently upholstered chairs (perhaps you have some in your basement from your last renovation), and a banner from an instant sign franchise.

You can be up and running practically overnight with your application zone. Get your haircolor department up and producing right away. Then you can reinvest some of the profits into upgrading!

The Consultation Zone

Ideally, consultations take place in a specially designed area. I am a firm believer that every salon guest ought to receive a consultation and be offered a variety of service options.

Before we delve into describing the layout of the consultation area, let's be straightforward about the nature of

"A color department, coupled with automatic consultations, really advances the goal of creating more impulse purchasing of color services."

consultation and clear up some common misconceptions surrounding its art and practice.

First, a consultation is not a brainstorming session or a free association idea exchange. "How about this?" "Have you tried that?" These are not confident or effective ways to advocate specific services or treatments. You are the expert, not the client. Be prepared to step up and advocate a specific course of action.

Second, the consultation is not primarily a discussion about hair length around the ears or about the neck. Surprisingly, this is what passes for consultation in many salons. The fact is that the haircut appointment has already purchased the haircut. Move the discussion to hair treatment and color. Extra service creates more benefit for the client and additional income for you.

Third, the consultation is not performed in the reception area, at the backbar, or at the cutting station. Realistically, some salons are in rather tight quarters and so sometimes this cannot be avoided. Ideally, though, salons should create and reserve a specific defined area for consultation with well-thought-out lighting, mirrors, and service merchandising elements. It is surprising that some stylists still opt to consult at their cutting chairs even in salons where a consultation area has been created. That is a serious mistake.

The practice of merely escorting guests to the cutting station and carrying on a conversation about desired hair length simply is not adequate. It will neither generate a substantial ticket nor distinguish you as a designer of high caliber. The idea is to move away from all the consultation emphasis on the haircut and move toward designing an entire look that includes coloring and perhaps texture.

A special consultation area sets the stage and communicates to guests that they have arrived somewhere that specializes in doing makeovers.

Ideally, the consultation area should be positioned so that the consultation mirrors clearly reflect all the excitement and showmanship that is taking place in the haircolor application zone. I recommend that after a salon tour and visit to the change room we let guests linger uninterrupted in the consultation zone for a moment or two to take in the whole show before their own consultation begins. They will automatically grow more interested in and confident about your haircolor talents with all this activity going on around them. The layout itself prepares the client psychologically to purchase haircolor on impulse.

Again, the consultation zone can be created overnight. You only need three things: chairs or stools for clients to sit on; mirrors; small shelves or holders for exhibits. Depending on the size of your salon you might have two, three, four, or five consultation stations lined up in a row. Hang a sign that says "Design Consultation" over the area, and you are in business.

> A primary aim of consultations is to stimulate additional purchasing. Consultations that focus on haircuts are fruitless. The guest has already bought the haircut.

An alternative approach would be to convert a cutting station or two into a consultation area. Half the salons I visit have empty stations that could be transformed into a consultation zone. Keep in mind that if you decide to do this, you must make sure that you carefully select and position the stations you are going to use. Strategically refine how they look in order to distinguish them from the ordinary cutting stations. Nevertheless, the first option is preferred if at all possible.

The Formulation Zone

The formulation room is the third key zone. This is where your magic formulas are fashioned. It needs to appear to be more than a dingy, dimly lit, converted closet.

As it is viewed from the consultation and application areas, the formulation zone needs to have a defined and appealing presence. An awning, special moldings, or even a neon sign at the point of entrance can help. Also, a distinctive curtain, drape, or other doorway design element can dramatically enhance the profile of your formulation zone.

How you enter and exit the formulation room ought to be thought out. Here is one place you can add an extra element of showmanship and bravado to the haircolor process. Even something as simple as a special cart upon which you wheel all your tools and foils and brushes can add entertainment value. Think of exciting formulation or mixing procedures you can do chairside to add excitement. Think of what they do in restaurants with Caesar Salads or Cherries Jubilee. Have some signature procedures and practices that completely distinguish you and your salon from everyone else.

Some Final Thoughts on Creating Your Haircolor Department

At the dawn of the Age of Retail back in 1970, salons did not have retail areas. If they had any retail products at all, they were generally kept under lock and key in a glass case for display. Of course today there is hardly a salon designed without a lot of consideration given to the retail area. In fact, there are entire businesses that do nothing more than sell salon retail products, as controversial as that has been. And we will see more of it.

Salon educators have mentioned creating a haircolor department for some time without getting very specific or at best making it seem like a complicated affair. Well, as you now know, it is simple and easy.

During the Age of Color, salons are going to be creating haircolor departments. It is already happening. A few haircolor salons are positioning themselves as market leaders right now. Move quickly. Time and again the first ones to market cream the business and enjoy the big windfall. Now is the time to situate yourself effectively for the Age of Haircolor, so move ahead boldly to be among the very first in your market area to strongly feature haircolor.

CONCLUSION

Every starting point through the five golden formulas is to determine where you are right now. If you want to achieve dramatic financial growth in your haircolor income, then calculating these five measurements is not an option. It is a requirement. Plant your feet firmly on the ground where you are right now.

Before you proceed any further stop, review, and precisely determine exactly where you stand right now. Refer to the Haircolor Success Formula Status Sheet (Table 2-1, page 32) and simply fill in the blanks for your actual performance. To determine where you are, go back over the last 100 salon visitors. This gives you a broad and specific sampling of your current state of affairs. Once you have an accurate picture, you can firmly and precisely set specific goals and objectives to improve your performance. You want to make measurable progress in reasonable time and in all areas.

Say that your haircolor market penetration is just 7 percent right now. Why not set a goal of improving that to 10 percent over the next week and then 12 percent over the next two weeks and 15 percent in three weeks. Do the same thing with haircolor as a percentage of service income. If right now it's at 9 percent, try to boost it to 12 percent in one week, 15 percent for the second week, and 18 percent in three weeks.

You can use your Haircolor Success Formula Status Sheet (Table 2-1) to keep track of your progress over the next four weeks. Make a few photocopies before you go too far, because you need to make a habit of tracking your progress. Make a commitment to yourself to spend 15 minutes at the end of each week to evaluate your haircolor performance. Something about the practice of keeping track of the numbers seems to attract the results we want. It also alerts us to whether we are on target or missing the boat. This is a simple system that is easy to use and that gives a realistic read on how you are advancing toward your goals.

> **"Enlighten yourself as to where you exactly stand with your haircolor business. Only then will you be in a position to set specific, measurable, and meaningful goals for haircolor income growth."**

Haircolor can get the job done when it comes to building your personal prestige and fortune as a hair designer. Take the time right now to calculate where you are at and set goals for where you want to go. Keep track of your progress. It's the first step in "planning your work and working your plan!"

What's most exciting is not merely watching the numbers grow but also realizing that those numbers reflect actual service to actual people! This is real evidence that you are making a greater and greater contribution to others. Real personal and professional fulfillment lies here.

Creating a haircolor department need not be an idea to wait on any longer. Now is the time to move. If you want to, you can literally have your haircolor department up and running in 24 hours. You can fine-tune your layout and presentation over time. The reality of a haircolor department in your salon is the fastest and surest way to assert your specialty and position your salon as the place for coloring in your community.

> *Here's what we discovered:*
> 1. *Haircolor specialization provides you with greater money-making power without limiting your options.*
> 2. *You can either package your entire salon as a haircoloring emporium or create a special haircolor department within your salon.*
> 3. *You are now fully aware of the three zones that make up you haircolor department: application, consultation, and formulation.*

Primary Haircolor Merchandising Tactics

A t the point of sale, there are a variety of ways you can proclaim haircoloring to salon guests. Point of sale refers to marketing and merchandising activity that occurs at the place of purchase. This is distinguished from advertising and marketing that takes place away from your business premises and that is ordinarily more focused on building salon traffic as well as market image and awareness. Now we review some of the fundamental methods you can use all the time to communicate your haircolor specialty at the point of purchase.

You'll discover "Primary Haircolor Merchandising Tactics" to help you enjoy more benefits from
1. using entry signage.
2. displaying model photos.
3. utilizing client photos.
4. exhibiting haircolor qualifications.
5. using manufacturers' promotional materials.
6. modeling color within the salon.

Using Entry Signage

Start communicating haircolor before patrons even walk through the salon door.

Your Main Sign

Be sure the main salon sign promotes your haircolor identity. As discussed previously, the very name of your salon, or a slogan attached to your name, needs to proclaim your haircolor specialty. Be sure this idea is carried through to your main business sign.

Your Entry Door

An eye-level sign right on your entryway door needs to communicate haircolor. You want first-time visitors to be confronted with the idea of haircoloring upon walking into your place of business. Whether it illustrates haircolor or contains your haircolor slogan, you want the door to communicate your haircolor specialty.

Use Basic Window Messages

Many salons make a list of their services in the front window. They include everything from children's cuts to bikini waxing to ear piercing. As a color specialty salon, you list your signature coloring services instead. Later on we review salon color menu development. You will ultimately develop several proprietary services worthy of special mention on your window.

Displaying Model Photos

Create a Color Feature Wall

Showcase photographs of beautifully haircolored models in a special area. Ideally these are your own hair models and the emphasis is clearly on the remarkable haircolor work your design team produces. Make it a fashion showcase that visitors can dependably reference to see what is current.

Keep It Current!

Change your photographs seasonally. A common error is for salons to do a set of photos and then keep those same model photos up on the walls for years. Out-of-date pictures dramatically decrease the effectiveness of your fashion wall. As a trendsetter, you want to show the new seasonal colors and designs in a beautifully framed, large color format.

Have Photographs of Your Best Work in Evidence throughout the Salon

Never underestimate this important concept. Strategically placed haircolor model photographs in the washroom, change room, consultation zone, and refreshment center serve to re-enforce the reality that you and your team are experts at haircoloring. That you show the initiative to design and display your fashionable color designs distinguishes you.

Utilizing Client Photos

Use Before and After Photos

Haircoloring plays beautifully into the before and after makeover photo. This tactic is perhaps the most tried and true method in the beauty business. Before and after photos never go out of style. Like a black dress or a blue blazer, before and after examples are fundamental, they are classic, and they work dependably! A 1990s business called Glamour Shots was completely based on the before and after idea.

Feature average salon clients transformed. Show the transformative value of your color work on Jane Q. Public. Not only can you use the before and after transformations in promotional material, you can also make photo albums full of makeovers. Keep these albums in the reception area and at other spots where guests linger. Illustrate both dramatic and subtle changes. Without turning off those who might prefer a modest change, be sure to also appeal to those who want a more exciting and daring transformation. Help salon guests relate and dream!

Have a Client Wall

Create an area to showcase snapshots of everyday clients with ravishing haircolor. You could mount these photos on a cork board in the change room, in the washroom, along a hallway, under glass at the reception desk, or in the waiting area. Imagine, hundreds of smiling faces, all with fresh haircolor, and all looking like the woman next door. This communicates the message that haircolor is not just for pretty young models. Haircolor is for everybody!

These basic approaches have been preached for years. Yet right now less than 10 percent of salons are working with these ideas in any meaningful way—not surprisingly, the 10 percent who are prospering. Our objective is not to re-invent the wheel. Yes, add a new twist, add a little creativity and imagination to your photos. Great! But use them! These are all fundamental strategies, and they work.

Exhibiting Haircolor Qualifications

Proudly display your notices and distinctions.

Create Automatic Authority with Diplomas

A simple piece of paper can make you appear to be an expert. This is one of the reasons professional offices typically exhibit academic certificates. A lot of the distributors and manufacturers offer advanced training opportunities and provide certificates of participation to those who attend. Whenever someone attends one of my live seminars, they walk away with a diploma. These need to be displayed. Simply taping them up on the station mirror is not satisfactory. Have them framed. Mount them to the wall in a strategic location such as the consultation zone. Their presence makes your recommendations more influential.

Assert Your Mastery with Trophies, Plaques, and Other Citations

Entering contests and winning awards for your work as a color designer builds value. A discreetly positioned awards case can add a lot of shine to your reputation.

Utilize Press Clippings

Actively pursue media coverage; then frame and display meaningful profiles. You also might want to frame and prominently display photos of your work that have been published.

Using Manufacturers' Promotional Materials

Place Materials Strategically

Posters, pamphlets, style books, and other point-of-sale materials are readily available from color producers. These can provide excellent resource material to help with fundamental salon merchandising.

The change room can be a particularly effective place to bombard your clients with strong haircolor messages. Depending on the price and value statement you want to make, you could literally wallpaper the change room with manufacturer posters. Or you could use a much softer approach and have only one or two elements discreetly positioned. The washroom could be an excellent spot to put manufacturers' haircolor literature for people to read. You have got a captive audience! Also, you could dry mount color company posters and place them in your salon window or on an easel that people see immediately upon entering your salon.

You Can Make the Manufacturer Part of Your Positioning

How extensively you want to rely on manufacturer support material depends a lot on your market and what you are trying to accomplish. I personally am a big believer in partnering with a key distributor and color manufacturer and adding powerful brand identity to the specific color used in the salon. On the other hand, a lot of successful color emporiums down-play the color brand completely and instead emphasize themselves as the focal point. Perhaps a blend of the two perspectives gives you the best of both. So, if you want to identify your salon with a particular color brand, do it cohesively and elegantly to make it part of your unique selling proposition.

Imagine Positioning Your Salon as a Haircolor Supermarket

There is a powerful merchandising option that has not yet been fully explored with haircolor. Just as some salons offer most or all major brands of wet lines, so too that some salons will position themselves to offer most or all brands of professional haircolor.

Those who advertise "All brands available" can create a very strong selling proposition. They can advertise a more comprehensive, sophisticated, and artistically advanced color service. This universal offering concept may blow you away. With the nature of coloring, it is difficult to imagine a salon mastering each and every major brand offering. But wait and see whether this prediction doesn't come to pass!

Another thing to look out for is salons retailing home color preparations, meaning salon stores that will begin to make professional brands of haircolor available to the public for home use. In fact, some haircolor lines may be developed purely for the purpose of salon retailing.

Be aware that in a general way this is already happening. On a limited scale, it happens through beauty stores, some of which claim to be professional only but wink and sell so-called professional haircoloring to the public. Today, the more exclusive brands are generally not available to the public through these outlets—not yet, anyway. For better or worse, I predict the day will come when they will be. Mergers and acquisitions we have seen make this clear to me. This is part of the dynamic and changing business landscape that unfolds before us. Simply be aware of what will happen so that you are not caught blind.

Colleagues, I am not making any value judgement on the merit of this inevitable development, but remember that you heard it here first. However, for a variety of reasons this development does not necessarily bode poorly for those who position and educate themselves as color specialists. A powerful reality is the value of your artistry and excellence and the comfort of the salon experience itself. Plus, most of the public will not enjoy satisfactory results with home experimentation and will inevitably come to the salon for haircolor services anyway.

Modeling Color Within the Salon

Make a Personal Fashion Statement, including Haircolor

Because hair fashion is the product, the physical appearance of everyone working in the salon must reinforce the merchandising strategy. Today, no hair fashion is complete without color. Everyone—male and female—who works in the salon must wear fresh, seasonal, contemporary color in their hair. The correct message is that color makes the look. You must be a product of what you are selling to experience maximum success. Your enthusiasm about color must start with your own personal statement.

Model the Latest Color Fashions

Make wearing color part of your merchandising strategy. Cooperatively plan who is going to wear which current shade so that as a team you showcase all the latest offerings. This modeling of color creates interest, builds desire, and helps persuade existing color clients to try something new, different, and perhaps more expensive. Just as with clothing, the latest color fashions can command a premium price point.

Consider a Special Uniform

Another strategy is to wear apparel that bolsters credibility for color. This can be something as simple as a badge that says Master Colorist, to embroidering Haircolor Technician on white lab coats used by colorists when they apply haircolor. Costume yourself and your team in a way that asserts haircolor expertise.

CONCLUSION

To everyone's eye, you want to create the powerful impression that your salon is first and foremost a haircoloring emporium. Everything from outside signage, to window displays, to feature photos must communicate HAIRCOLOR!

Using these basic visual merchandising strategies will go a long way toward creating automatic confidence in your haircolor expertise and help set the stage for impulse purchasing of haircolor.

Here is what we learned:

1. *You can put haircolor on the agenda with your outside signage.*
2. *You can use photos of salon models to boost your credibility with color.*
3. *Photos of happy color clients dramatize your expertise with commercial looks that satisfy.*
4. *You can create extra confidence by displaying your educational credentials openly.*
5. *Branded materials are a great source of merchandising muscle.*
6. *Always be your own best color advertisement by being a product of the product.*

Printing Your Haircolor Identity

I f you want to make the really big money during the Age of Haircolor, you must boldly assert your salon identity as a haircoloring establishment and yourself as a haircolor specialist. Every printed item you use and circulate to existing and potential salon clients must sing haircolor.

In "Printing Your Haircolor Identity," you learn ways to get added haircolor positioning power out of everyday salon printed materials, including:
1. your business cards.
2. your gift certificates.
3. your retention and referral materials.
4. your newsletters.
5. your postcard mailings.

Your Business Cards

Everyone must have a business card that includes name, salon name, complete address including postal code, as well as the phone number with area code. If you have a fax, e-mail or Web site, put that on your card too. That's basic. To transform your card into a haircolor promotional device, there is more to consider. (See Figure 4-1.)

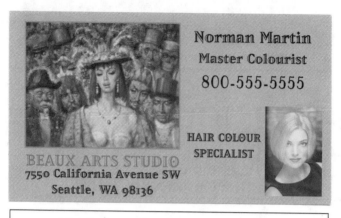

FIGURE 4-1. Sample business card

Remember The Slogan

Put a tag slogan after the name of your salon that says something like, "The Haircolor Specialists" or "Your Place for Haircolor."

Give Yourself a Title

Use a title like Master Colorist or Haircolor Director to communicate your expertise. Place that title right under your name. Simply declare yourself expert and print it on your card. There is now a designation you can receive for haircolor mastery. If and when you establish official credentials, have that printed on your card. Another powerful specialty worth declaring on the business card is "Color Correction Specialist."

List Your Haircoloring Services on Your Card

To help people understand that you design complete looks, mention "Designer Color & Cut" or "Same Day Color and Perm."

Make an Offer

You could make a universal offer such as, "Discover your best shades. Experience a complimentary color consultation. Call for your courtesy appointment."

Your Business Card Can Be Improved by Going Full Color

Feature a glamorously finished salon haircolor model. Find a printer in your area who does picture cards for real estate agents. These printers often gang print a dozen or more card jobs on a single sheet. Consequently, they can offer a very favorable price. Going full color will say "color" and make a powerful positioning statement. It's hard to say "color" in black and white!

Your Gift Certificates

Gift certificates are among the most powerful promotional devices you ever use. There are two kinds: The ones you donate or give away, and the ones you sell. In either case, always keep this rule: Haircolor must comprise part of the service that the recipient gets. (See Figure 4-2.)

Gift Certificates as Donations

If you donate a haircut and style for a charity door prize, be sure to include color and emphasize haircolor as the most valuable component of them all. Always communicate the idea that no visit is complete without color. Get the prize winner thinking color. Further, because color is part of the giveaway, shouldn't it be part of the consultation? How about color services that go beyond what was won?

Also, because you include color when you donate a service, doesn't it naturally follow that you should include color when people are paying for your design expertise? This kind of thinking helps staff to

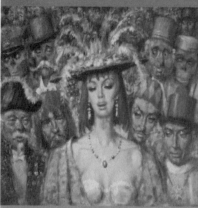
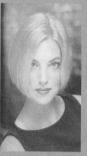
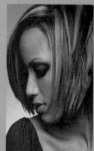

A GIFT FOR YOU...A GIFT FOR YOU...A GIFT FOR YOU...

HAIR FASHION

BEAUX ARTS STUDIO

7550 California Ave. SW
Seattle, WA 98136 • 800-555-5555

HAIR COLOUR
SPECIALIST

*Reserve Your Appointment
Call Now 800-555-5555*

GIFT CERTIFICATE

ACCEPT YOUR INVITATION FOR A
COMPLIMENTARY
PROFESSIONAL HAIRCOLOURING SERVICE

Choose from...

• colour staining

• colour express

• topcoat colour

• glossing

*Call **800-555-5555** now
for your appointment time!*

BEAUX ARTS STUDIO
7550 California Ave. SW
Seattle, WA 98136

PRESORTED
STANDARD
US POSTAGE PAID
SEATTLE, WA
PERMIT NO. 1685

Please notify us if you are planning to
redeem your gift certificate at the time
of your appointment. You must be at
least 21 years of age. First time guest
only, please. Please call *800-555-5555*
for your appointment. Limited Time Offer.

FIGURE 4-2. Sample gift certificate. (*Insert photos provided by Scruples Professional Salon Products, Inc. [left] and Clairol Professional Hair Products [right].*)

see color as a natural component of the design process. Also, it gives a tremendous boost to the credibility and feel of your consultations.

Gift Certificates as Gifts

You can sell thousands and thousands of dollars worth of gift certificates to your existing clients that can be presented as gifts to brides, co-workers, family, friends, and many others. Rather than make your gift certificates for a plain dollar amount, make them for a package of services. The "Color Me Beautiful Makeover Afternoon" gift is more saleable gift than a plain $100 gift certificate.

Remember, make sure that the gift certificates themselves shout color by their very design. You could use a colorful envelope, make a colorful statement or slogan on the certificate itself, and use color in the very names of the service packages themselves.

Your Retention and Referral Materials

Plant the Color Seed Early with Referrals

A special referral card, including an incentive, is a good idea. For example, make your incentive a complimentary color analysis. A lot of salons prefer to avoid making an offer that discounts. Rather than offer a discount, give away a consultation. This way you get the first time visitor thinking haircolor. It also gives you full opportunity to freely discuss color options during the consultation. The idea here is that you keep color the focus everywhere.

Reward Referral Sources with Color

Many salons reward clients who refer new visitors. Rather than give away a free haircut, reward with a gift certificate for a complimentary color-oriented service. Perhaps a color rinse or a color enhancing shampoo or conditioning treatment. Color, color everywhere!

Reward Loyalty with Color

If a customer is still with you by the time a birthday or anniversary date comes, you have cause for celebration. Acknowledge the occasion with color. If you have a frequent visitor or purchaser program, make color the premium reward.

Be sure all your printed materials here keep with the color message. "Paint the town. It's your birthday. May it be your most colorful one yet!" That could be the tag line in your birthday card accompanied by a gift certificate for color.

One frequent user program, for example, rewarded patrons who had spent $500 in a year on products and services with a complimentary $50 color service. The guests had to keep track of their own receipts. The owner reported that the promotion was their most successful and effortless reward program ever. Develop a brochure and give it a colorful title—for example, "Reward Yourself with Every Color under the Rainbow!"

Your Newsletters

Make It a Color Newsletter

Your newsletter mailing to your clients can be all about color. Summarize or write your own articles that promote color. Each newsletter should talk about some aspect of color and emphasize the design advice, service, and products you provide.

Use Full-Color Pictures and Colorful Screens throughout Your Newsletter

If you have a list of several thousand patrons, you can probably produce a full-color 11 x 17 folded newsletter and have it delivered for under a dollar per client. Do that four times a year and stay in touch with your customers annually for $4 a head. Keep in mind this may be less than one tenth what it could cost to get a fresh guest in the door the first time. Remember that it is always easier to sell more to your existing clientele than to try to recruit new ones.

Make It a Self-Mailer

Making your newsletter a self-mailer eliminates the need to place it in an envelope. This both reduces costs and increases effectiveness. Also, everyone at the post office gets a read, and your immediate impact on the client recipient is heightened.

Your Postcard Mailings

Use Postcards

The most effective form of salon direct marketing to the house list is the postcard. There is no envelope to open! You convey an immediate message. Research shows that postcards are more widely read by recipients than letters. They simply work better.

Many salon communications, including thank you cards and reminder cards, can take place easily and effectively by postcard. Make sure you use a separate look for each type of card. Also, consider oversized postcards, which have more impact. Double-check current postal regulations to see how large you can go without incurring undue postage expense.

Print Full Color

Give strong consideration to using full color postcards. Again, full color printing is the order of the day. This need not be a budget buster if you learn to purchase wisely. As with business cards, there are printers who make a business of postcards and prepare them at reasonable cost.

Consider Brand Cards

Talk to your distributor or haircolor manufacturer. Sometimes these sources have inventories of preprinted brand postcards you can access, often at little or no cost to you. Perhaps they may be willing to co-op a mailing if you use one of their images on the postcard. That is a good idea because their images have the big budget look and they can often provide you with color separations, keeping your production costs down.

CONCLUSION

You can re-invent practically all of your printed materials to give them the haircolor spin. Remember, people tend to believe what they read, so make sure yours says haircolor!

Here's what we learned:
1. *Your business card establishes your authority and mastery as a haircolor specialist.*
2. *If you give anything away, give away haircolor.*
3. *Your salon newsletter need do no more than report on and sell advancements in haircolor at your salon.*
4. *Full-color printing is the order of the day, and with smart sourcing, you can build a colorful image without breaking the budget.*

5

Preparing Your Salon Menu

L ess than one in five salons has a menu. And less than one in twenty of those goes beyond the mere listing of available services and prices. Those are not menus; they are really just price lists.

Within a matter of years, menus will be common. Ultimately salon menus will be the most effective selling tool in use in salons. A salon menu that emphasizes color services is the most powerful print-ed positioning statement you can make. It distinguishes you at once.

In "Preparing Your Salon Menu," you learn about the following:

1. why a salon menu has value

2. what to include in your salon menu

3. how to package services and create proprietary offerings

4. how to appeal to different economic levels and demographic groups

5. how to produce a menu inexpensively

Why a Salon Menu Has Value

An effective salon menu is highly valuable to you because it will

- make you more money through stimulating impulse purchasing of unplanned services and home maintenance products.

- be a very effective tool in providing more influential consultations.

- serve as a take-home memento for current salon guests, helping client retention.

- stimulate referral activity because of its pass-along feature and because it can be designed to pre-sell potential clients and invite them to the salon.

- distinguish you from other salons in the market that do not have an effective menu.

- be a highly powerful direct mail and direct marketing tool to existing or prospective clients.

- create additional walk-in traffic by tastefully positioning your menu outside—much like a restaurant.

- enable you to market 24 hours a day by keeping a supply of your menus available to the public in a permanent holder situated immediately outside your salon.

- be a wonderful promotional tool you can distribute at special events, gatherings, or presentations.

- enhance staff morale and retention.

> Your salon menu is the most powerful point-of-sale marketing tool you have.

The salon menu is an item whose time has come. Few salons have yet developed a menu. Those that have generally can benefit from considerable improvement. So whether you have a menu or not, the following pointers teach you how to make your first menu or how to make your existing menu considerably better.

What to Include in Your Salon Menu

The Basics

Everything that you should have on your business card you should have on your menu: your salon name; your complete address including city, state or province, and postal code; your phone number and area code; fax, e-mail, or Web site, if applicable. You might consider a small map pointing out your exact location.

It is a good idea to put your salon mission statement on the menu. Hopefully you have one! It could be something like, "Dedicated to offering the finest image and color design services for fashion conscious patrons in the tri-state area"—or even something considerably longer! Perhaps a statement on the history or philosophy of the salon would be of value. A photo of the salon owner or the salon team would be appropriate as well.

Your Guarantee

A guarantee of satisfaction is a very positive element to include—it creates confidence among patrons. It conveys authority and demonstrates confidence in your work. Increased purchasing will be directly attributable to your guarantee. In the event a client is dissatisfied, a guarantee will open free communication which will enable you to immediately remedy the problem and thus retain the client.

Here is an example of a guarantee:

Your Double Satisfaction Guarantee:
We are so confident you will be absolutely delighted with the color and styling work you receive from our design team that we offer you an iron-clad double guarantee of satisfaction as follows:
1. *If you are unhappy the day of the service, let us know right away and we will correct it on the spot at no additional charge.*
2. *Wear the color and design for a full fourteen days. If it does not completely live up to your expectations of quality and longevity—or if for any reason whatsoever you are dissatisfied—simply let us know and we will immediately schedule an appointment for you so that we can adjust the color or style to your satisfaction. Your pleasure and satisfaction is our purpose!*

Your guarantee enables you to stimulate significantly more impulse haircolor purchasing. This fact more than outweighs the occasional nuisance (as opposed to a legitimate claim) that may result. The fact is that you guarantee your services anyway. Make that a potent selling point and confidence booster in your menu.

Have faith in the good will and integrity of people. If it happens at all that someone would take unfair advantage of your guarantee, it would be so rare an occurrence as to be barely worth talking about. True, you may be taken advantage of at some time. If a client abuses your guarantee, simply refund them their money and wish them better luck elsewhere.

The Description of Services

First, you should be clear about what not to do. Salons that have a menu frequently list their haircolor services like this:

Color Services

Permanent Haircolor	$ _____
Semi-Permanent Haircolor	$ _____
Demi-Permanent Haircolor	$ _____
Highlights	
• Foil Method	$ _____
• Cap Method	$ _____
Bleaching	$ _____
Double Process Coloring	$ _____

Doing it this way does not work. It simply is not an effective way to position color properly. There is no image building, no creating desire, and no stimulating of purchases. These are technical descriptions that often have little or no meaning to the consumer, especially the consumer who has never worn coloring. Further, this kind of terminology makes haircolor seem like a commodity. That is an impression you want to avoid.

In summary, your menu includes all the basic elements, your guarantee, and your description of services. Now, let's dig a little further.

How to Package Services and Create Proprietary Offerings

You want to romance the idea of haircoloring, arouse interest, distinguish the color services in your salon, and stimulate a "Why not try it?" impulse ordering mood. By way of overview, the goal is to create a consumer friendly menu that lists and describes all your salon offerings in an appealing way that will command attention, arouse desire, and stimulate purchasing.

To do this, we package services. In packaging services, it is important to keep in mind the value of offering variety. The goal is to offer a wide assortment of services that will appeal to key segments of the market. Let everyone feel that they have an appropriate and exciting color service to order. Also, you may want to distinguish

> **"The goal is to package a wide assortment of color services that will appeal to key segments of the market."**

your color services from those available elsewhere by packaging signature and proprietary offerings. That is power!

Divide Services into Categories or Headings

Think of a restaurant menu for a moment. The customer is presented with choices for appetizers, soups and salads, main courses, desserts, and beverages. Some menus might divide main courses into chicken, fish, beef, pork, pasta, and the like. Many give these headings appealing titles. Rather than fish, they call it "Fruits of the Sea." These are the same principles you should follow in creating categories for your services.

Consider the major divisions under which you will offer specific services. There are general categories and special categories. Special categories can include things like special combined service packages, gift certificate offerings, and home maintenance systems. Some special categories may emphasize services to a specific demographic category like "Gentlemen's Grooming" or "Ethnic Glamour." (Special categories are discussed more later.)

Although haircolor is your specialty, you will probably find it valuable to include other general categories of service like "Precision Haircutting and Styling" and "Healthy Hair Treatments" and "Body Building and Texturizing Systems."

When it comes to haircolor, go all out. You will divide haircolor into a number of different service category headings. You will want creative names for what the industry calls "permanent color," "semi-permanent color," "highlights," "double process coloring," "designer coloring," and so on. (I suggest some creative ideas later.)

Fashion-Specific Service Offerings

You want to be aware of four ideas in packaging specific service offerings. Once reviewed, you have the practical information necessary to design service offerings capable of virtually selling themselves. The four concepts are the following:

1. *the principle of differentiation*
2. *the principle of segmentation*
3. *the naming of services*
4. *the formula of menu copyrighting*

THE PRINCIPLE OF DIFFERENTIATION

Find ways to distinguish one haircolor service from another and then package those distinctions. To package and market haircolor like a commodity is a mistake.

Take for example the scene in the movie *Forest Gump* when Bubba explained to Forest the variety of ways shrimp could be prepared: fried, baked, boiled, broiled, stewed, chilled, barbecued. You could use a whole variety of different sauces and additives and spices. And if you were to go into a shrimp restaurant in Gulfport, Mississippi, they would probably have 20 different ways they could prepare and serve shrimp. Furthermore, the prices would be all over the place. Peel and eat would be one price, and Shrimp Creole would be another. Size would have an impact. Even with something as simple as shrimp, they figured out a lot of ways to segment the product to justify different price points as well as add interest and variety. They could simply say "Shrimp" just as some salons say "Haircolor," but they would be missing the principle of differentiation.

Let's look at permanent haircolor as a case in point. Think about various technical procedures you can use to differentiate permanent haircolor services.

- Contemplate the variety of equipment you can employ.
- Consider the different additives you can use.
- Think about different formulations you could use.
- Consider different ways you can mix and blend ingredients.
- Contemplate that, within brands, there are different families of permanent haircolor.
- Recognize that you can offer to perform a permanent color service with regular, upgraded, or premium color brands or formulations.

These elements are your keys to product differentiation. With a little bit of imagination, permanent haircolor can be differentiated into a half dozen or more distinguishable services.

> Recognize that you can use the variety of procedures, techniques, equipment, and formulations available to differentiate one similar color service from another.

THE PRINCIPLE OF SEGMENTATION

Find ways to position haircolor services to appeal to different segments of the market. As was mentioned previously, some segments— for example, men—may be sufficiently special as to warrant their own category of services. But under your general categories, be aware that salon guests, though unique, fit into defined demographic and psychographic categories.

As mentioned previously, demographics is the study of measurable statistics in a population such as age, gender, income, occupation, size of family, and the like. Psychographics is the study of measurable statistics of how members of a population behave. Knowing who your market is demographically and understanding how they are likely to behave psychographically can be very powerful information when deciding how to package haircolor service offerings for maximum success.

Consider psychographics, the newer discipline. It asks questions about what matters to people and what is likely to stimulate their behavior in predictable ways. Their lifestyles and preferences are going to impact what they elect to buy. So, ask yourself, "What kind of a message do I need to communicate surrounding haircolor to arouse the values and affections of my target market?" Then, reflect these values in your menu and service packaging.

Consider you own market area and the values that are held deeply by the people you want as customers. What people value in Las Vegas may be different from what people value in Laguna Beach or in Peoria. Your challenge is to make sure that your service offerings reflect the values that psychologically appeal to the market you want to attract. And, as a professional in the fashion business, do not merely reflect—LEAD!

Depending on the size of your market, you can wrap yourself completely around one psychological theme. But many of you will want to position offerings that reflect the values and behaviors of several groups. For example, you may have a permanent haircolor service positioned for the youth market, another for the working woman market, another for the executive woman, one for the homemaker, and one for the senior citizen. Of course, under your gentlemen's grooming services, you could offer a permanent haircolor service or two. If you do not want all these age groups and lifestyles in your salon, you can simply exclude them by purposely avoiding service offerings that would appeal to them. Remember, you are under no obligation to be all things to all people.

THE NAMING OF SERVICES

With the principles of differentiation and segmentation firmly in mind, you want to develop a family of service names that have appeal, that have a thread of consistency, and that imply a key benefit.

Being able to incorporate a deeply emotional implied benefit in the name of your services is particularly powerful. The benefits of prestige, recognition, romance, safety, security, love, success, and acceptance, and the rich variety of words and images that evoke these special feelings need to be artfully integrated into the very names of service products. At this point do not worry about the names of specific shades or colors. Create the names of services that will be color customized for each client.

Unless one has a death wish, it seems automatic that one would want service names that would be appealing to the target market. Consistency among service names is a great way to accomplish this. Salons need to establish some sort of a theme that can act as inspiration for their various service names. Such a theme should be broad enough to provide lots of possibilities. Remember, we're not talking about color collections or color names now, we're talking about service names.

Geographical locations are one possibility. Local or regional landmarks or exotic international spots could be an inspiration. If your salon is in a big city, you could use landmarks in your town. For example:

SERVICE CATEGORY: Permanently a New Yorker

SPECIFIC OFFERINGS: Wall Street Wonder
Fashion Avenue Flair
Times Square Tawdry
East Side Ego
Chelsea Cheers
Greenwich Village Vamp
Broadway Bombshell

Notice how the names are designed to appeal to specific market segments and how they carry an implied image benefit. Notice also, that these services are non–color-specific so that you have the freedom to customize the color for each guest. And remember that what distinguishes one offering from the others is the equipment used, the additives employed, the application method, and so on.

You could use a European idea:

SERVICE CATEGORY: Semi-Permanent Visits to
                      Colorful Europe

SPECIFIC OFFERINGS: An Afternoon in Paris
                      Italian Wanderings
                      Swiss Delight
                      Roman Romance
                      Swedish Express
                      Mediterranean Moods
                      Monte Carlo Royale

You could use a regional theme:

SERVICE CATEGORY: Highlights of Southern Charm

SPECIFIC OFFERINGS: Charleston Chunks
                      Savannah Streaks
                      Tennessee Twists
                      Blue Ridge Lights
                      Florida Strands
                      Dimensions of Atlanta

The plain fact is that you can use birds, fish, fruits, flowers, foods, furs, animals, vegetables, motion pictures, foreign words and expressions, natural elements, weather conditions, famous artists, fashion designers, design themes, Broadway shows, famous songs, famous personalities . . . you can use just about any theme your heart desires!

Humor can also be brought into play when naming services. But it must be done carefully. If your menu features categories, names, and descriptions that have an entertainment value, buying becomes more fun for clients and sales go up accordingly. However, humor is difficult to pull off effectively. There is always the potential that someone can be offended. Writing humor is serious work, so if you are going to attempt a humorous menu, take advantage of outside consultation and even use a focus group to make sure it works.

The Formula of Menu Copyrighting: The Name of the Service Attracts Attention; The Copy Sells It for You

Think of being in a fine restaurant. Open the menu and you see a display of dishes under a variety of interesting categories. Under each category you are able to contemplate all the possibilities for your pleasure.

Take appetizers for example. You often find eight or ten or more appetizer selections. Beneath or next to each appetizer offering there is a description that has a tremendous influence on which appetizer, if any, you select. The menu description ultimately sells the item. If none of the descriptions appeals to you, you order none. If one looks good, you get it. Consider the influence of descriptive copy on these options:

> *Shrimp Cocktail*
> **$6.95**

or

> ## Jumbo Shrimp Cocktail Provençale
> *Eight mouthwatering, plump, and tender—absolutely fresh—*
> *Jumbo Shrimp. Your taste buds will delight with each bite.*
> *Delicately spiced to bring out the full flavor. Served with our own*
> *custom-blended cocktail sauce—made with a European flair.*
> *Or, ask your server about other delicious sauce possibilities.*
> *Treat yourself to our house specialty!*
> **$6.95**

Which one are you more likely to order?

There are two things to remember about menu descriptions. First, they are read. Many people will spend several minutes looking over a menu very carefully and reading each and every word—often several times—when considering what to order. The copy makes the sale.

Second, the menu prompts questions. An alert server knows that the customer's question is a powerful buying signal. A little reassurance and recommendation will probably result in an impulse purchase.

That's why a little hook prompting the reader to ask for further details is such a great way to promote impulse purchase choices.

The description—the copy—makes the sale or at the very least sets the sale up! There is a direct link between the name and descriptive copy about a menu item and the amount of purchasing the item attracts.

One very straightforward way to sell services in your salon menu is to use the problem/solution structure. Your clients will understand it, you will find it easy to work with, and you will appreciate that it provides a simplicity and consistency to all the offering descriptions. I use the following formula when creating a menu entry for a service:

> Solution (name of service)
> 1. Problem solved
> 2. Practical benefit expressed
> 3. Point of distinction
> 4. Psychological value achieved
> 5. Secondary benefit

For example:

> *Color Textures:* Your flat hair days are over! Experience incredible fullness, body, and control accompanied by vibrant shine with no-perm Color Textures. A special additive is introduced into your color formulation that prompts extra thickness and volume that lasts and lasts. You add confidence to your appearance and give your presence and style a positive lift. Custom blended to secure the exact shade that is you.

Notice all the elements in the example and how they work together:

> Solution (name of service)——*Color Textures*
> 1. Problem solved—Your flat hair days are over!

2. Practical benefit expressed—Experience incredible fullness, body, and control accompanied by vibrant shine with no-perm Color Textures.

3. Point of distinction—A special additive is introduced into your color formulation that prompts extra thickness and volume that lasts and lasts.

4. Psychological value achieved—You add confidence to your appearance and give your presence and style a positive lift.

5. Secondary benefit—Custom blended to secure the exact shade that is you.

Notice how the menu merely hints at the technical details, procedures, formulas, or chemistry in its point of distinction. Benefit-oriented copy is all you want in the menu.

Designers must be prepared to elaborate on descriptive details: "What exactly is the special additive?" "How do you blend it in?" "How does it work?" "Will it dry out my hair?" "Will it affect the color?" Script, practice, and role-play these interactions to make them as smooth as silk. Those questions are buying signals. Make sure you strike while the iron is hot!

How to Appeal to Different Economic Levels and Demographic Groups

Pricing your services is an important strategic decision. On the one hand you don't want to give the service away and on the other hand, you don't want to scare away perspective clients. My recommendation is to offer some lead-in pricing and then up-sell into more elaborate and expensive coloring and other add-on service and product offerings.

You Must State Your Prices

Just as with retail products, you must be very specific about the prices of your color and other services. You must communicate your prices clearly. Many of you will feel perfectly comfortable about printing your prices right in your menu and you should. Others may feel unsure because of planned price adjustments in the near term. Under those circumstances you may elect to have a separately printed insert to communicate pricing.

Avoid "up" pricing: "$40.00 & up" is the price. This kind of pricing discourages impulse purchasing and patron questioning. It creates fear. It is not consumer friendly. Consider the menu item that says, "Lobster—Market Price". You can't sell much lobster that way! Now, if you wish, you can certainly put a small fine-print disclaimer in an inconspicuous spot on the menu communicating that prices may vary due to the length, texture, or condition of hair at the discretion of the salon. Check with your lawyer to make sure that any disclaimer you decide to use meets legal specifications. But remember, the "up" strategy simply does not work, so avoid it!

Offer a Lead-in Color Service

One of the real benefits of haircoloring is that you can start someone off with a basic service and then gradually upgrade to more and more expensive services. Be sure your menu takes advantage of this reality.

For example, offer a signature color service at a relatively modest price point to entice new patrons into the color arena. It could be something as simple as a color shampoo service, a color conditioner, or a basic semi-permanent color blend which can be applied quickly and that entertains the client with a fun and painless color experience. The strategy is to build from there on future visits.

Use Sliding Scale Pricing on the Same Procedures

You can offer a variety of price points that escalate according to the experience, seniority, or expertise of the designer doing the work.

The length of hair being short, medium, or long can be a stated price variable. (See Figure 5-1.)

Another way to offer a variety of price points is to offer a few different brands or qualities of haircolor. Put a dollar or two between the

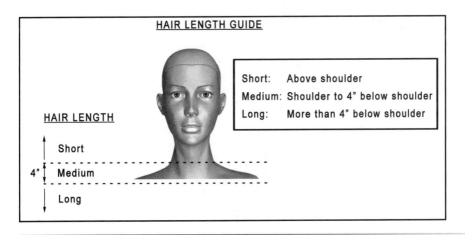

FIGURE 5-1. Sample hair length price chart

price of the various brands or lines you offer. In my seminars, I always recommend premium pricing the latest color shade options released by your color manufacturer. Always sell exclusivity for a premium.

Highlighting services can be differentiated by the amount of hair that is highlighted—a third, a half, or a full head. An illustration of this would answer a lot of questions. (See Figure 5-2.)

Highlight Options

Coverage	_1/3_	_1/2_	_Full_
Jr. Colorist	$25	$35	$45
Colorist	$35	$50	$70
Sr. Colorist	$45	$55	$75
Master	$55	$70	$90

Select our deluxe brand color for only $4 extra or treat yourself to the very best premium color for only $7.50 more.
Aren't you worth it?!

This table is for illustration purposes only to see how you might incorporate a variety of pricing levels into highlighting, as an example.

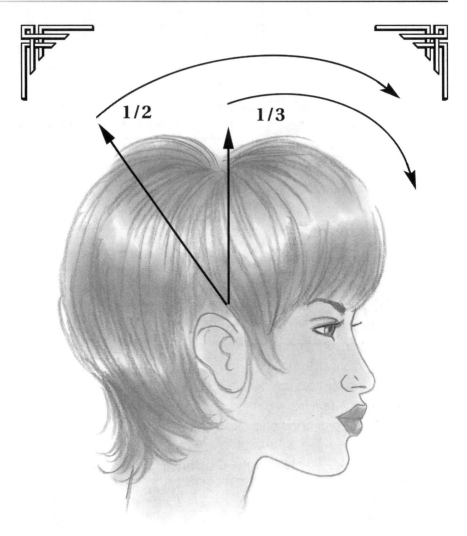

Colourist
1/3 - $35, 1/2 - $50, full - $70
Master Colourist
1/3 - $45, 1/2 - $60, full - $80

FIGURE 5-2. Sample highlight price chart

Notice how a patron can start for as little as $25 and then move up to as much as $62.50 for the exact same thing by choosing a Master colorist and premium color for the service.

Other factors affecting your pricing options include the designers you have on staff, your market area, the population your serve, your level of business, prevailing prices in your community, and the image you are trying to project in the marketplace.

Also note that a simple graph can be used to communicate pricing for multiple options within a service category.

Vary Price by Service Offering

Of course another strategy is to differentiate price by service offering. That makes a lot of sense because of how you differentiate services within a category. Say you have six different permanent color options. Each could have a different price. Some might be the same price. Plus, you can always vary price within a service offering by distinguishing elements such as length of hair and designer status.

Combine Elements to Achieve Higher Tickets

Another effective pricing strategy is to combine basic services into a complete package. Give your patrons the option of purchasing à la carte or full service. Do what McDonald's did. The Full Meal Deal brings together the sandwich, potato, and beverage. McDonald's discovered that too many patrons were skipping one of the three elements, resulting in lower ticket averages. By combining items, they solved the problem.

Start with a new, basic hairstyle package and include services that many patrons might otherwise skip. Two great ones are the signature color service already discussed, as well as the upgraded conditioning treatment. In my view we must include haircolor as part of the basic service package. Currently the basic package is wash, cut, and style. We must add color to that.

> **"Re-invent your basic hair service package to include color."**

If the guest does not want the color, make the wash, cut, and style separate à la carte services. If you want to be real bold you could price those separate items so that it costs more for them separately than it would to buy the basic service package that includes your signature color service. Some patrons will be smart and attempt to buy the package and tell you to hold the color. Your response must be that without the color, the other services are strictly à la carte.

Now, you might argue that this will discourage your haircut customers who do not want coloring. The response is "That's great." You win both ways. You wind up with more money from your haircut only clients who choose to stay. Those who leave create more room for clients who will buy haircolor—which is your target market anyway!

Your treatment services need to be integrated into the menu and revenue stream.

1. As it stands, virtually 100 percent of treatments provided in salons are done so at no charge.

2. The reasons are:
   a. The hairstylist is afraid to ask for the money.
   b. The service has not been packaged.
   c. The service has not been presented in consultation.
   d. The service has no showbiz performance delivery elements.

Packaging, Presentation, Performance

3. Using the principles learned here, name and package six or eight treatment services designed to deal with the recurring problems people have with their hair, such as dryness, oiliness, dandruff, static, split ends, unmanageability, hair loss, protein loss, moisture imbalance, cuticle layer damage, and problems with elasticity.

4. Price treatments from $2.00 to $20.00 or more, keeping them well within the range of impulse purchasing.

You may want to consider introducing a new basic service offering that includes the following elements:

- Your basic signature introductory color service
- Shampoo service
- Selected hair "treatment" service
- Precision haircut
- Finished style

Grouping these elements together allows you to offer "the works" pricing and introduce a lot of reluctant patrons to haircolor as part of your standard full service hair offering. Further, this also helps surround your treatment services with higher perceived value.

By reinventing your basic service offering, you accomplish several important goals.

- You increase the average ticket.
- You entice a larger percentage of your guests into haircolor.
- You are in a position to upgrade the color sale in the future.
- You have attached a specific value to your treatment services.
- You should be able to sell more of those treatments individually on future visits.

Offer Service Packages

In addition to the basic hair design package just described, your menu is also an excellent place to sell a large assortment of upgraded service packages. The more services you have to offer at your salon, the larger the variety of packages you can create and market.

An entire page or panel of your menu could be devoted to service packages. Some full service salons and many day and destination spas have been on the bandwagon with these beauty offerings for some time. Many day spas have five, or ten, or even more half-day, full-day, and series packages that they make available to visitors. When done properly, this has a sensational impact on cash flow. These packages are typically priced at over $100.00 and can run into several hundred dollars. Obviously, color has to be included in this mix.

Color-only packages work well in the salon. A color-only package consists of putting all your color services together. You can include ideas like color draping and even wardrobe consultation to go along with the nails, hair, and makeup to create a harmonious, well-tailored look.

You should include color services in all your planned or existing packages. Highlight the color value and weave the color idea into the name of the package. For example, transform a "Bride's Day of Beauty" to "The Blushing Bride's Colorful Day of Beauty" and add some color service enhancements to the package.

Promote Gift Certificates

You want to have a Gift Certificate heading in your menu that is noticeably supported with other point-of-sale signage, display, and literature. Some salons offer dollar-denominated gift certificates. You will discover that package gift certificates work better. Service packages make wonderful gifts! Develop an attractive gift box or elaborate envelope for your gift certificate. It could be very effective to illustrate someone giving and receiving one of your gift certificates in your menu to dramatize the effect.

You might enhance the value of your gift certificates by offering a delivery service. Your service could offer singing telegrams, or your delivery person could wear a costume appropriate to the occasion and bearing your logo. You might offer a small gift to the purchaser during times when gift certificate sales are brisk, like December, Mother's Day, Valentine's Day, Administrative Professional's Day, and the like. Use your menu to sell gift certificates.

Use "Create Your Own" Packages to Increase Spending

Another packaging idea that can work effectively is to let patrons select one service from three or four headings. This has the effect of offering selection while at the same time stimulating the use of extra services. This can be a great program to use because the designer can get involved and advise what combination of service options works best for the client during their consultation. For example:

Hair Treats	_Permanent Solutions_	_Highlight Your Style_	_Afterthoughts_
Select I	Select I	Select I	Select I
Treat I	Color I	Highlight I	Nails I
Treat 2	Color 2	Highlight 2	Nails 2
Treat 3	Color 3	Highlight 3	Make-up I
Treat 4	Color 4	Highlight 4	Make-up 2

Notice: No haircut and style. Certainly, those elements could be included if you wished. Or they could be offered separately at an extra price. You could offer a two-tiered price for your haircut and style as well: one regular price if purchased à la carte; another perhaps slightly lower price if purchased in combination with the "create your own" package.

Package Home Maintenance Items with Services

You can include retail and home maintenance offerings into packages. This can be done in a very simple or a more elaborate way. For example, you could have five levels of service, with names that indicate increasingly higher levels:

1. Signature Color—the basic no-frills color

2. Bronze Signature Color—color with cut and style

3. Silver Signature Color—color, highlight, treatment, cut, and style

4. Gold Signature Color—color, highlight, treatment, cut, and style with take-home custom color blended shampoo and conditioner

5. Platinum Signature Color—color, highlight, treatment, cut, and style with take-home custom color blended shampoo and conditioner, styling lotion, spray and gloss, and a gift certificate good for a future visit

This idea can be taken a step further into client retention strategies. Offer upgrade certificates, called "color miles," that frequent visitors could accumulate and use to move from one class of service to a more premium class. But that's for later discussion.

Incorporate Special Offers to Stimulate More Spending

Let's return to the restaurant example. Most restaurants offer specials of the day. Sometimes these are attached to the menu. Ideally, the server, well rehearsed, describes the chef's special preparations in intimate, mouthwatering detail. Patrons give undivided attention to the discussion of the specials. Keep in mind that these dishes are often premium priced.

A common communication error is to confuse the word special with the word discount. Specials can relate more to rareness, exclusivity, or occasion. Keep this in mind.

> A special need not be value-priced. It can be a seasonal or special occasion or late breaking fashion offering that in fact commands premium dollars.

Develop a dozen or more service specials that run the whole gamut of service categories. And be on the constant lookout for new ideas that come along. Keep in mind the principles of packaging, presentation, and performance.

On a regular rotation basis, roll out your specials of the day, week, or month. Time them to coincide with changing seasons and holidays. Make a big deal out of them. Some of these specials could become a tradition at your salon. Charge well for them. Up-sell them on the phone when people are booking appointments. Sell them at the greeting desk. Sell them on a menu attachment. Sell them during the consultation in the same way the restaurant server would describe the special menu additions. Amaze yourself with how many patrons will say, "Yes."

How to Produce a Menu Inexpensively

There are so many advantages and opportunities with a salon menu that you are probably anxious to get yours going right away. Be aware that you can develop some side menus and description brochures apart from your regular menu.

Consider, for example, a special menu for treatments. If you have custom blended or private labeled products, then a menu or brochure could be appropriate. For some of the more popular, special, or expensive propositions, you may want to develop an additional leaflet with more details. Particular service packages may warrant this kind of special treatment. Additionally, you could develop a brochure applauding the overall virtues of color and explaining how your color services accessorize the client for a cohesive look ideal for today's fashion requirements.

A full-color salon menu can really create a powerful haircolor image. You can use it numerous ways to cement your salon's position and build sales. There are four ways you can produce your menu.

Custom Print a Large Quantity of Full-Color Menus

This choice really only makes sense if your salon is doing at least several hundred thousand dollars of business per year. Plan on a $10,000 budget, although you could do it for $5,000.

You need several people. First, you need salon models for the photographs you will reproduce. You could use manufacturer supplied photos of models if you have a very strong allegiance to a particular color brand and want to benefit from their marketing of a particular image. But, if that's not the case, you need your own models.

Next, locate a knowledgable menu copywriter and designer. Find an expert to fine-tune your menu concept (I make myself available for this work). An experienced professional can substantially refine a presentation and dramatically enhance response. Dollars spent on experienced outside marketing expertise is money well spent. Knowing where you can source expert consultation is a definite competitive advantage.

Third, identify a graphic designer who has the skill and ability to make good use of full color printing capabilities. Starting immediately, become an observer of quality color printed items that appear in your community. Find out where the artwork was done. But be aware that graphic artists are not marketers, and rarely do they have more than a passing awareness of marketing principles. Try not to rely on them too much for advice. Rather, identify a good graphic designer who can execute your ideas with some sparkle and panache and who is a perfectionist. Graphic designers charge over a wide range for their services: One will accept $200, but another wants $2,000. Remember that price is not always an indicator of quality.

Fourth, find a printer who can get a high-quality job done on time and at a fair price. Perhaps you already have a relationship with a printer. That's a good place to start. Keep in mind that printers are often specialists. Do not use your printer just because that would be convenient. Look at recently printed samples of comparable quality work. Make sure that the printer is not outsourcing the full-color printing. Consider alternatives. Always deal with the source. Cut out any go-betweens and salespeople. Go straight to the president of the printing company. These firms are often small, so it should be quite easy. Position yourself as a house account. Then compare prices. Cheapest does not equal best. Use your gut feeling about who can deliver quality and stand behind the work. Delivery on a timely basis can be quite the issue with printers.

When getting quotes, make sure that you compare exact specifications. Quantity, paper, number of color separations, and other variables need to be held constant so that you can do an accurate comparison.

Think about paper. Choose a paper stock that is appropriate—something like a white coated card stock. You could consider going to a 100 pound coated white paper stock. Stay away from anything less than 80 pound because you want your menu to have a feeling of substance. Sometimes printers buy particular papers in a large quantity or have some stock sitting in inventory that they can sharpen their pencils on. Consider these possibilities. However, do not under any circumstances agree to an inferior or inappropriate paper stock to save a few dollars. Unless you have a lot of experience with printing, be conservative with your paper choice. Avoid textured, linen, laid, or any exotic papers. Those textures just do not print color well. Examine a wide range of printed samples to judge for yourself.

Your printer will encourage you to print a larger quantity to benefit from a lower per unit cost. It's a good idea to keep your quantities modest to start with because the day your menus are delivered, you will see things you will want to change for the next time. You may go through three or four printings before you get exactly what you want long term. That is when you can print your lifetime supply!

> **"To start, print a modest quantity of your menu. You will want the opportunity to fine-tune your menu without having to trash a large quantity."**

Custom Design a Small Number of Deluxe Salon Menus

Thousands of custom printed full-color menus is a costly proposition. This is not appropriate for smaller salon operations or booth renters. So by using full-color photocopying technology, you can create exactly the number of menus you require. Also, if you know your way around computers, you can use a scanner and full-color printer to get the job done.

To give your menu a deluxe look, use attractive leather binders. Look around some fancy stationery stores and get the leather binders you want to use. For a price, these can be embossed with your salon logo, though that is not completely necessary.

You will make full-color menu pages. You can use a separate page for each menu category. Think of an 8- or 10-page Chinese menu with one page for the chow mein and another for the pork, the beef, the chicken, and the fried rice. You can develop a page for each salon service category: one for treatments, another for textures, and several more for each category of color service. You can incorporate all the elements we talked about before. If you or someone you know can do page making on the computer, you are home free. But do not hesitate to have a graphics person create beautiful consistent page layouts and help you to incorporate haircolor model photos or illustrations. Use full-color photographs of salon models wearing the color styles you describe. Use all the packaging, pricing, and copy techniques you have learned here.

Then, simply run off the number of menus you need, dry mount or laminate the pages, and assemble them in your leather binders. Because you are making a small number of them, your total budget need not be more than a few hundred dollars at absolute most. You could probably make one or two for under $100!

You get all the point-of-sale benefits from this kind of menu that the larger operations get with their mass produced efforts. You can place a couple copies in your reception area, one in your washroom, and a couple in your consultation area. Make anywhere from 2 to 20 copies. This will work great!

The main drawback here is that you cannot really give these menus away. So, their use as a retention or referral tool is lost. You will not be able to direct mail them. But perhaps one of the following ideas can bridge this gap for you.

Use Preprinted Shells

You can obtain preprinted shells that are designed for you to complete with your own information. These are available at better office supply stores and via mail order. They are preprinted with border art and contain significant empty space for you to insert your message. These shells are designed to be run through a laser printer or a photocopier. So, once you have your message designed, you can copy a quantity of 20 or 50 or 100. Shells can perhaps be best used for supplementary or specialty menus.

With a color ink-jet printer you can add additional custom color photo imagery. Because this is more complicated, you should work with someone who has experience using this kind of equipment. To date, color photocopiers require special papers and if you're going to go to the expense of color photocopying, you need not have the extra expense of shells because you can have page maker software design your own borders and give you a custom look. The cost-effectiveness of these methods will improve over time.

Looking to the future, as menu development becomes standard in the salon profession, you will find that some manufacturers will be more likely to develop brand shells that can be customized as menus.

Consider Cooperative Direct Mail

Another way to get a low-cost full-color menu is to do a menu distribution with a cooperative direct mailing company. In a lot of areas and for a lot of markets these companies continue to produce meaningful measurable results. Although the days of being able to build your business on the back of this kind of distribution seem to be over, this method can still be effective if used selectively.

These companies work with you to design and print a variety of full-color sheet sizes and options, which they distribute to your immediate area. They have professional quality graphic design capability. They put together 8½ x 11-inch restaurant menus by the thousands, so their in-house designers have unusually broad experience at menu layout. And, in addition to your own photos, they have access to substantial libraries of full-color fashion photos you can use.

They give you automatic distribution of your menu. They encourage you to make some kind of offer so that you can measure results of your efforts. But that does not mean that you have to go to a coupon look.

Finally—the clincher—they give you a small stack of overruns, which you can have laid down on card stock and laminated to use as an in-salon menu. Two for the price of one, so to speak. You should be starting getting the idea that you can afford full color if you use your imagination.

CONCLUSION

You now have a whole arsenal of ways that you can position yourself and your salon for haircoloring. By using these strategies you will create automatic authority and communicate your expertise with haircoloring. Your menu does all this and more.

The time to move along with your salon menu is right now. As a color salon, your message is "We do haircoloring, and we also cut and treat and wave your hair to create a true designer look." Your menu enables you to communicate that most effectively.

Here is what we have learned:

1. *A salon menu offers powerful marketing and selling advantages.*
2. *Your menu benefits from your mission statement and satisfaction guarantee.*
3. *You package your services so that they are consumer friendly, and you emphasize the practical and psychological benefits that appeal to segments of the population.*
4. *You can price your services specifically while showing a great deal of latitude at the same time.*
5. *You can produce a menu inexpensively.*

Promoting Haircolor Profitably

P romotions are commercial tools to compel consumers to act or think in certain ways. Any promotion without a call to action is incomplete. There are a variety of promotional ways and means to dramatically enhance haircolor income. The strategies you decide to use depend on the goals you plan to achieve. It is therefore essential to first clearly determine your promotional objectives. As Steven Covey wrote in *The Seven Habits of Highly Effective People*, "begin with the end in mind."

> In "Promoting Haircolor Profitably," you get a better under-
> standing of the financial tools and dynamics associated with
> professional haircoloring. You discover:
>
> 1. the goal of increasing haircolor market penetration with cur-
>   rent salon clients.
> 2. the goal of upgrading current color clients to more expensive
>   color service packages.
> 3. the goal of attracting fresh new color customers to your
>   salon.
> 4. the goal of improving home maintenance sales to color
>   clients.
> 5. the goal of retaining haircolor clients.
> 6. the measurable results *principle of promotions.*

The Goal of Increasing Haircolor Market Penetration with Current Salon Clients

The first potential goal of a haircolor promotion is to entice more existing clients into the professional haircolor arena. In Chapter 2 we discussed haircolor market penetration and learned how to calculate haircolor market penetration by determining what percentage of current clients are purchasing haircolor services.

Here the goal is to increase that percentage and improve haircolor market penetration. Specifically the objective is to convert first-time clients and clients who are home color users to haircoloring in professional salons.

The Lifetime Value of a Haircolor Client

Increasing haircolor market penetration is worth the effort. Consider the lifetime value of a haircolor customer. The lifetime value concept focuses on recognizing the amount of money a customer will spend over the life of your professional relationship.

> **"Haircolor can boost spending by up to $2,000 or more over the average lifetime of a salon client. Multiply that by a few hundred clients!"**

It stands to reason that haircolor clients will spend at least two to three times as much as non–haircolor clients over the average life of the relationship, probably more. First, haircolor is a great loyalty service, so it is likely that the average life span of a color client is greater than that for clients in general. Second, the extra money color clients spend on services and home maintenance items significantly adds up over time. On a single visit an extra $30 or $40 may not seem like much in the scheme of things. But if you multiply that by ten visits a year, over an average traditional client relationship of four and a half years, the reality of haircolor can boost spending by up to $2,000 or more over the average lifetime of a salon client. Multiply that by a few hundred clients and you are talking about the extra cash necessary to enable you to retire in style. Is the effort worth it to you?

Understanding New Client Cost

Sophisticated marketers recognize that they have to invest to increase market share. There is a cost in time, effort, and funds. Look at this investment as your new client cost. And you can get very specific about calculating new client cost by comparing the amount invested in a particular marketing campaign with the amount of actual new clients it produces.

The lowest new client cost is usually the one associated with selling something more to an existing patron. This means that your existing noncolor customers are your best prospects to become color clients. This is not only because of the relationship you have already established with them, but also because it is financially efficient.

With existing salon clients, you are able to avoid traffic-building client attraction marketing and advertising costs. Also, existing customers generally convert to the new haircolor sale at a greater rate than do other prospects. It stands to reason that a maximum amount of effort ought to be applied to converting existing salon clients to professional haircoloring.

The Goal of Upgrading Current Color Clients to More Expensive Color Service Packages

A second major goal would be to up-sell current color clients. It bears repeating that being able to upgrade clients is one of the real beauties of haircolor. Color clients can be enticed into more expensive color services with relative ease.

As you can imagine, this objective requires a completely different set of promotional techniques to accomplish than the ones you need to entice clients into the color arena to begin with.

Instead of calculating haircolor market penetration figures, you will be more interested in calculating the growth in the average color ticket and the growth in the average number of color services per client, both of which were discussed in Chapter 2.

Packaging, Presentation, and Performance

Thoughtful packaging of services will enable you to upgrade client spending. You may unveil a series of designer coloring services that are more technically and artistically sophisticated. Those are worth premium money. Or you may have some special high fashion or seasonal offerings that can command a bigger ticket. Do not forget about packaging a treatment with the color to move clients into more expensive visits.

Two, three, and four color services on the same head is a worthy idea! Make sure your seasonal signature looks require several steps so that you can attach a high dollar value to them. Even if it is technically simple, make sure that you emphasize packaging, presentation, and performance strategies capable of adding enough value to achieve higher spending for your artistic concept and accomplishment.

Use Your Artistic Reputation to Justify Higher Pricing

In apparel, a classic black dress or blue blazer can be had for under $100 or for several hundred dollars depending on the fabric, cut, style, workmanship, and designer. The designer is often the most important variable in moving up price.

You are the designer of each and every look you create. You personally perform it, or you oversee the performance of it. You have positioned yourself as a foremost colorist. These facts need to be packaged as an incredible value for the client so that you have the opportunity to charge for them.

Pursue Added Client Spending Enthusiastically

Do not be afraid of moving your clients through progressively higher and higher spending thresholds. Whether that barrier be $20, $40, $100, or even $200, you want to periodically give clients a good reason to step up to the next level. Recognize that price barriers get farther and farther apart as you get more and more expensive! The fact is that many salon patrons link price with quality and will be attracted to higher-priced services. A promotion with the objective of increasing haircolor client spending must be designed to address these opportunities.

Consumer behavior research reveals that price is only one of several vital factors considered when making a purchase decision. Other factors are typically more influential, particularly in the fashion and personal appearance arena. There are so many self-esteem issues tied into fashion and appearance. The cost of our services is so very low in comparison to the psychological value we can deliver. The price levels typically commanded at salons are already undervalued.

Consider the amounts people spend at restaurants and show performances, which are only fleeting experiences, and you can begin to see the value we deliver in more relative terms. Prestige, recognition, acceptance, beauty, fashion, glamor,

> Two, three, and four color services on the same head is a worthy idea!

success, happiness, and self-confidence are only some of the benefits we deliver—and the benefits linger. That value merits a fair price tag in the marketplace.

The Quality, Service, Price Dynamic

Think of it like this. Three main factors are involved in the delivery of any product or service: quality, service, and price. The adage is that when it comes to quality, service, and price, consumers can pick any two. If they want outstanding service and excellent quality, then they have to pay the price. If price is the only consideration, then they either sacrifice quality or service—and frequently both.

My personal read is that once people get to a certain age, perhaps in their mid-30s to early 40s, and have reached a basic level of comfort and stability in their life, then quality and service become more important than price. This is certainly true when dealing with the prime demographic and psychographic group of people in their best earning years who are active and involved and participate fully in life. In my opinion the bulk of baby boomers are not highly price sensitive when it comes to their personal appearance services. Consequently, there is real opportunity to move them into progressively more and more spending on color services.

Promotions Provide Consumers with the Logical Reasons to Make Emotional Decisions

Consumers make most buying decisions for purely emotional reasons. However, people like to justify emotional actions with logic. This is where your promotional activity comes into play. Promotions provide the logical justification for emotional decisions. That is why you never have to give away the store when your goal is to upgrade existing color clients. You have to provide just enough reason for the consumer to logically justify what is essentially an emotional and impulsive decision. No more, no less. Further, that is why in the promotional strategies discussed here we focus completely on low-cost premiums rather than costly price discounts, which are very counterproductive to the bottom line. It is better to include something extra that costs $0.50 than make a discount of $5.00!

The Goal of Attracting Fresh Color Customers to Your Salon

Attracting fresh color clients to your salon is the third major goal to consider. Positioned as a haircolor specialist, you will want to engage in ongoing promotional strategies designed to bring new color-oriented clients your way. Up to this point, goals have surrounded yielding more business from existing patrons. Now, for the first time the goal is finding new business in the marketplace.

New Client Cost Revisited

Marketing costs are associated with attracting new customers through the door. There is a cost in time, energy, and money to generate new business. Generally, the more time and effort put forth, the less money spent.

However, neither time nor effort nor funds guarantee results. Experienced professionals know that it is definitely possible to spend a lot of money and expend a lot of effort and still come up empty-handed. Thus the concept of new client cost, which provides us with objective criteria to compare the results of different promotional activity and expenditures. Some efforts work better than others, and this analysis helps us determine which ones are most financially worthwhile. Naturally the highest yielding efforts bear repeating and expanding.

Paying attention to new client cost means specifically measuring the results of each promotional activity. Those results are compared to the cost of the promotion to determine whether it was profitable. Start looking at each promotion as a test. Here is some of the data you need to collect surrounding each specific promotional effort.

Cost per Inquiry

How many phone calls (making an appointment or not) or walk-ins were generated specifically by the promotion? For example, a $500 ad that generated 25 phone calls would have a $20 cost per inquiry (500 / 25 = 20).

> **Cost of promotion ÷ Total inquiries generated =
> Cost per inquiry**

Cost per Visit

How many people visited as a result of the promotion? For example, of the 25 people who called from the $500 ad, only 10 actually made a visit, yielding a $50 cost per visit (500 / 10 = 50).

> **Cost of promotion ÷ Total visits generated =
> Cost per visit**

Cost per Sale

How many people bought as a result of the promotion? For example, of the 10 who visited as a result of the $500 ad, 8 bought, yielding a cost per sale of $62.50 (500 / 8 = 62.50).

> **Cost of promotion ÷ Total number of sales =
> Cost per sale**

TOTAL YIELD

How much was purchased as a direct result of the promotion? For example, the ticket values were all over the place. One got away with a $10 bang trim and another with a $12 treatment; but five of them had coloring, and three of them spent over $100. In total they spent $640.

> Total sales dollars = Total yield

YIELD PER SALE

How much did they buy in services on average? For example, the eight spent a total of $640, resulting in an average ticket of $80 (640 / 8 = 80).

> Total sales dollars ÷ Total number of sales = Yield per sale

SURPLUS/DEFICIT

Did we make or lose money? For example, total sales less cost of promotion equals surplus or deficit. The cost of the promotion was $500 yielding sales of $640 and creating a surplus of $140 (640 − 500 = 140).

> Total sales dollars − Cost of promotion = Surplus or (Deficit)

SURPLUS/DEFICIT PER SALE

How much did we make or lose per sale? For example, yield per sale less cost per sale equals surplus or deficit per sale. Each sale averaged an $80 yield against a $62.50 promotional cost, creating a surplus of $17.50 per sale (80 − 62.50 = 17.50).

> Surplus or (Deficit) ÷ Total number of sales =
> Surplus or (Deficit) per sale

Table 6-1 presents a summary of all these investment return calculations.

Table 6-1		Haircolor Promotional Investment Return Sheet

		FORMULA	*RESULTS*
Marketing Investment	#1	Count $	
Total Inquiries	#2	Count #	
Cost per Inquiry	#3	#1 / #2 = #3 *Answer is $*	
Total Visits	#4	Count #	
Cost per Visit	#5	#1 / #4 = #5 *Answer is $*	
Total Number Sold	#6	Count #	
Cost per Sale	#7	#1 / #6 = #7 *Answer is $*	
Total Yield Services	#8	Count $	
Service Yield per Sale	#9	#8 / #6 = #9 *Answer is $*	
Total Yield Retail	#10	Count $	
Retail Yield per Sale	#11	#10 / #6 = #11 *Answer is $*	
Total Yield	#12	Count $	
Total Yield Surplus or Deficit	#13	#12 – #1 = #13 *Answer is $*	
Surplus or Deficit per Sale	#14	#13 / #6 = #14 *Answer is $*	

Understanding Delivery Costs

How much does it cost to deliver one additional service in your salon, on average? These are what we would call incremental delivery costs. Incremental delivery costs are those costs that you can specifically relate to delivering service to the new client. You are already paying for electricity, rent, water, telephone, reception, and a host of other costs whether that one new person visits or not. The concern here is the extra specific cost attributable to delivering service to that guest. These service delivery costs fall into the categories of payroll and product.

Payroll Delivery Costs

Salon management can choose from a variety of pay systems. If a salon is on a straight commission pay system, management could well pay out 50 percent of service revenues or more in labor costs just to deliver an extra service. On the other hand, if a salon uses a straight salary or hourly pay system, then the cost of labor directly attributable to delivering the extra service could be negligible.

Product Delivery Costs

Calculating product delivery costs for services is pretty straightforward. An accountant would think of it as cost of goods sold. That is, in terms of the goods being used, how much does it cost to deliver a service?

If a $30 jug of shampoo does 120 shampoos, then it costs $0.25 per shampoo. If some services require two or three shampoos, you add them up. If a tube or bottle of color costs $3 per application, then that's what it is. If a multi-application service requires that you open several bottles or tubes, then add them all up. Computer programs are available that keep track of how many feet of cotton and how many ounces of toner and developer are used.

You may discover that you spend $1 in product to deliver a $20 cut and style and $5 in product to deliver a $50 service including color and $12 in product to deliver a $100 service package. In this example we spent $1 + $5 + $12 = $18. We yielded $20 + $50 + $100 = $170.

Here is the calculation: Total dollar yield divided by total product delivery cost calculates product delivery cost as a percentage of service sales.

In this case $170 / $18 = 9.44 percent. To simplify the calculations, round it up to 10 percent. Often the higher the ticket, the higher the product delivery cost. So, in coming up with an average that we can apply across the board, 10 percent is a good conservative yardstick for our example.

> Sourcing supplies economically can reduce product delivery costs by 30 percent to 50 percent—savings that improve both margins and profits.

Depending on how good you are at sourcing supplies, your product delivery cost could be higher or it could be considerably less. Naturally, your service pricing levels also have an impact. Make your own calculations and determine the product delivery costs for your salon as a percentage of your service ticket. Come up with an average to apply across the board.

Now you can be more precise and calculate the product delivery costs directly associated with each salon service. Make it a project for 8 to 12 weeks to track and link all these product delivery expenses on a service-by-service basis. Then calculate product delivery costs as a percentage of each service. If the scope of your operation warrants that depth of analysis, do it.

Determining Profit per Sale

Calculating new client cost and service delivery costs helps us determine profit per sale. In the previous example, the $500 promotion created 8 new customers who spent an average of $80 a head creating a surplus of $17.50 each. If the product delivery cost was 10 percent of the $80 that each spent, then it would average $8 per new customer. Subtracting the $8 product delivery cost from the $17.50 surplus leaves $9.50 profit per new guest.

As you can imagine, your pay system becomes extremely pivotal in determining whether or not you actually make a profit on this first visit. If you pay 50 percent of the $80 ticket in labor costs, you are into a serious deficit. If you pay $8 an hour and the visits averaged an hour, then you are still ahead by $1.50, which is just under 2 percent of the average ticket.

Anytime you can be in the plus territory at all on a guest's first visit, you are winning. Often you may have to be content with just avoiding a deficit when comparing yield to your cost of promotion. Covering product delivery costs on the first ticket is wonderful, and covering payroll delivery costs on the first ticket is fantastic.

The main thing to focus on is the lifetime value of the client. The costs associated with client retention and your other re-sell promotional investments will be marginal when compared to new client costs, so your profit opportunity is significantly more lucrative on subsequent visits. Plus, when you add retail sales margins and low-cost referral prospecting to the lifetime value of your new client, then you can really be ahead of the game.

The Goal of Improving Home Maintenance Sales to Color Clients

The fourth major goal is retail sales to haircolor clients. Naturally you want your color patrons to be on your home maintenance system. Haircolor will continue to be a very positive development when it comes to salon retailing for two reasons. First, color clients are more likely to buy retail products than are noncolor clients. They have invested in a look that needs maintenance, and they generally are people who care about their day-to-day appearance.

Second, there are more retail products for the color client today than ever before. Specialty retail products have been introduced specifically for home maintenance support for the color client. Salons can now custom blend color shampoos and conditioners. Many color hair cosmetic preparations have been introduced, such as color infused shampoos and conditioners as well as color enriched mousses and other fixatives. Finishing products that simply make the color look brighter and shinier are now available. This has been a very dynamic area for salon retailing. All this indicates that many professionals expect the salon color client to be a major retail purchaser. Other than the development of product offerings for men, color has been one of the few bright spots in salon retailing for quite a few years now.

> **"Generally color clients will demand and purchase more retail products than others. Improving your color business automatically improves your retail sales."**

There are four main objectives you can track with haircolor client retail purchasing. A discussion of each follows.

Color Retail to Color Service Ratio

This is the classic calculation salons have been tracking for some time now. The rule of thumb has been that for every $1.00 of service, you should sell $0.25 of retail—a 25 percent retail to service ratio. You simply divide retail sales by service sales to calculate this percentage. For example, $200 in retail sales divided by $1,000 in service sales equals .2 or 20 percent.

To calculate this, add up all the service purchases and retail purchases made by guests who had color. Then divide retail sales to color clients by service sales to color clients to determine retail sales as a percentage of service sales for color clients. For example, $250 in retail sales to color clients divided by $1,000 in service sales to color clients equals .25 or 25 percent.

> Color retail purchases ÷ Color service purchases =
> Color retail to color service ratio

A number of factors influence the ability to accomplish this. Keep in mind that color service tickets are generally larger than average, which could put downward pressure on retail sales as a percentage of service sales. However, as we continue our analysis you could well find a link associating higher service tickets and higher average retail sales. Also, if the goal is to increase the retail to service ratio for color clients, we would want to make sure that we were not doing that at the expense of the average size of service tickets. The catch-22 is that steady retail sales in the face of declining service sales will show a statistical improvement in the retail to service ratio. Yet, that is not what we are looking for. The preference is to see improvement in an environment of across-the-board sales.

Retail Market Penetration

This is another way of looking at market penetration from a retail point of view. Just as you can calculate what percentage of total salon clients purchase retail, so too you can calculate what percentage of salon color clients purchase retail. You may find it interesting to compare your overall retail market penetration with your color client retail market penetration to determine whether you have better retail market penetration among color clients. The best guess is that you do, which is encouraging.

Simply divide the color clients who bought retail by the total number of color clients to determine your retail market penetration with color clients. If 30 of the last 100 color clients purchased at least one retail item, then the retail market penetration with color clients is 30 / 100 = .3 or 30 percent.

> **Color clients with retail ÷ Total color clients =**
> **Retail market penetration**

If your goal is to increase that percentage, which is a worthy goal, initiate promotional activity geared toward having more of your salon color clients purchase home maintenance packages.

Retail Sales per Color Client

Look at the average amount spent by salon guest on retail items. If the last 100 salon guests spent a total of $500 on retail, then the average retail per guest would be $5.

Simply calculate the average retail ticket per color client. Divide the total retail purchases made by color clients by the total number of color clients to determine the average retail purchase made by a color client. For example, if you had 25 color clients visit during the time period who had purchased $500 in retail items, you would divide $500 by 25 to arrive at $20 in retail purchases by color clients.

**Total retail sales to color clients ÷ Total color clients =
Retail sales per color client**

Again, it would not be surprising if the average retail purchase for color clients was greater than for clients in general.

Average Retail Purchase Size

Here the concern is how much retail was purchased when a purchase was made. Continuing with the previous example, say that of the last 25 color guests only 10 purchased retail products. Now divide the $500 in retail sales by 10, and the average retail ticket is $50 ($500 / 10 = $50).

**Total retail sales to color clients ÷ Color clients buying retail =
Average retail purchase size**

Again, it would not be surprising if the average retail sale made to a color client was noticeably higher than a retail sale made to a non-color client. Sometimes, designers make the mistake of thinking that when people are spending a lot on services, they cannot afford to spend a lot on retail. My personal experience has been that the more they spend on service, the more they will spend on retail. Check it out for yourself.

Table 6-2 presents a summary of these home maintenance sales calculations.

Table 6-2   Home Maintenance Sales to Haircolor Clients Status Sheet

Retail Results for Total Salon Business		*FORMULA*	*RESULTS*	Retail Results for Color Business		*FORMULA*	*RESULTS*
Total Sales	#1	Count $		Total Sales to Color Guests	#1	Count $	
Service Sales	#2	Count $		Service Sales to Color Guests	#2	Count $	
Retail Sales	#3	Count $		Retail Sales to Color Guests	#3	Count $	
Total Guests	#4	Count #		Total Color Guests	#4	Count #	
Guests Purchasing Retail	#5	Count #		Color Guests Purchasing Retail	#5	Count #	
Ratio of Guests Purchasing Retail	#6	#5 / #4 = #6 *Answer is %*		Ratio of Color Guests Purchasing Retail	#6	#5 / #4 = #6 *Answer is %*	
Service/ Retail Ratio	#7	#3 / #2 = #7 *Answer is %*		Service/ Retail Ratio for Color Guests	#7	#3 / #2 = #7 *Answer is %*	
Retail per Guest	#8	#3 / #4 = #8 *Answer is $*		Retail per Color Guest	#8	#3 / #4 = #8 *Answer is $*	
Retail per Retail Guest	#9	#3 / #5 = #9 *Answer is $*		Retail per Retail Color Guest	#9	#3 / #5 = #9 *Answer is $*	

The Goal of Retaining Haircolor Clients

If we want to get the lifetime value of new client relationships, then we must retain clients. Client retention is the real sweetness of any promotional campaign. And it must be a central goal or you could just wind up spinning wheels.

Setting the stage for the additional visits and purchases is pivotal. The great pool hall player Minnesota Fats never made a shot without making sure the cue ball was in the right position to make the next shot. In fact, he usually thought many shots ahead. This mentality is what client retention is all about.

In the raw, client retention has to do with what percentage of first-time visitors become regular clients. A regular client is someone who has visited four or more times. Computer programs can track this for you.

Possible strategies on pursuing haircolor clients are discussed later in the book. For now, recognize that haircolor client retention must be an area of focus and must be thought about when designing promotions.

The *Measurable Results* Principle of Promotions

One of the key issues with meaningful goals is that they must meet the test of measurability. If you cannot calculate what is happening and gauge your progress with numbers, then it is not a good business goal. All five goal-setting areas discussed here meet this objective.

Here are the seven steps to use when implementing any promotion.

1. *Know where you are (calculated number).*
2. *Know where you want to go (projected number).*
3. *Plan how to get there.*
4. *Work your plan.*
5. *Make midstream adjustments and fine-tuning where necessary.*
6. *Calculate results (calculated number).*
7. *Evaluate results (comparison of numbers).*

Steps 1, 2, 6, and 7 all have to do with specific numerical analysis. To get the real power out of your promotion, you must get into the numbers. Make it an easy to follow system. Those with clearly defined goals and a well conceived plan of action are the ones making the money in this business. Those who are fascinated with seeing the numerical results are the ones who make the swiftest progress and enjoy the sweetest financial results.

CONCLUSION

Holding a sale to get some new color clients may be a common strategy, but it is likely to be a foolish one! Before conducting a color promotion, you have to be clear about what it is you are trying to accomplish. Then with the end in mind, you work backward to devise strategies that will advance your agenda.

You pick your promotional methods depending on what you are trying to accomplish. Ideally, you want to create promotions with some depth. You need to plan several moves ahead to solidify new client relationships. You have to be able to measure results so that you are not forced to merely speculate on the value of a promotion. Know your costs, track your results, and calculate your profits. That way you will be in a position to promote haircolor profitably.

Here is what we learned:
1. *You can increase haircolor market penetration with current salon clients.*
2. *You can upgrade current color clients to more expensive color service packages.*
3. *You can attract fresh new color customers to your salon.*
4. *You can improve home maintenance sales to color clients.*
5. *You can retain haircolor clients.*
6. *You can use the measurable results principle with haircolor promotional activity.*

Powerful Visual Merchandising of Haircolor

Visual merchandising can be defined as the practice of promoting purchases of goods and services through the use of visual prompting. Theoretically, there are limitless ways to create visual impressions capable of getting the job done. Truth be told, merchandising is an art!

Naturally, the haircoloring service you provide can be brought to market effectively or ineffectively. When you think about it, you are already a merchant of haircolor. You are merchandising right now. You are already making a statement about haircoloring in your salon. That is one of the things to be conscious of when it comes to merchandising—it is an automatic. Merchandising is not something you choose to do or not to do, it just happens. Right now, today, at this very minute you and your salon are making statements to clients and consumers about haircoloring. You are communicating your haircolor capabilities. You are communicating value and quality. You are communicating whether or not haircolor has a priority position at your salon. You are communicating perhaps more than you realize.

> **"Merchandising is not something you choose to do or not to do, it happens automatically."**

The problem is that salons and salon professionals all too often are not fully aware that they are communicating a message. Nor are they aware what their existing message communicates about value, quality, and service. In the consumer's mind, you are the image you put forth. This is not only true in terms of your personal presence; not only true in terms of your advertising and promotion; but also true in terms of messages you transmit at the point of sale. This is one of the areas of greatest opportunity in the salon profession.

Not understanding this opportunity often means that salons invest little or no effort into effective merchandising. If little or no thought goes into merchandising your color image, then you will not have much of a color image. The image that automatically gets presented will not do much to dramatize your expertise, artistry, or quality. If fact, your current merchandising message may be counterproductive to what you in fact want to communicate.

> In "Powerful Visual Merchandising of Haircolor" you discover:
> 1. how to use both image displays and buying displays to stimu-
>   late unplanned purchasing.
> 2. ways to masterfully display the exact image and message
>   you want to communicate.
> 3. how to use all the design elements that make displays
>   memorable and effective.
> 4. how to use signs more effectively.
> 5. the display zones in your salon and what works best for each.

How to Use Both Image Displays and Buying Displays to Stimulate Unplanned Purchasing

Recognize the difference between image display and buying display.

Buying Displays

Buying displays are specifically created to dispense merchandise. In the salon, buying displays are primarily used for retail items. The mere presentation of product is display. Naturally, elements can be added to enhance value and entice additional purchasing. The techniques of effective merchandise presentation to stimulate added buying are outside the scope of this book.

But consider a few important points.

THE RECOMMENDATION IS PRACTICALLY EVERYTHING

The clear and direct recommendation of the designer is the strongest variable in stimulating retail sales. Haircolor necessitates the need for the home maintenance recommendation. It must happen consistently and automatically.

HOME MAINTENANCE SYSTEMS RULE

Packaging several items together in a home maintenance system will stimulate extra purchasing because of the value perception. Packaging a system of three to six items together flows naturally into the most powerful retail offer of all—the gift with purchase. The consumer purchases a group of items and receives something extra "absolutely free." Have you noticed how this merchandising tool has become a mainstay at some emporiums?!

SECONDARY DISPLAYS MEAN SALES

Use secondary displays for featured product and product package offerings. Merely putting featured offerings on the shelf along with the other items is not nearly as effective as creating a secondary display in a high-traffic area for just that one product special. A haircolor month with a haircolor home maintenance package would be a natural for this.

THE LAW OF MARKETS

Show the product in massive abundance. Many salons waste time with the minimalist approach. Large volume need not be down market or give the drug store feel. The Law of Markets is a fundamental economic reality. Supply creates its own demand. The greater the supply, the greater the demand. Added inventory, on its own power, will increase purchasing.

Dress Up Your Buying Displays

Add supporting elements like props, posters, signs, and other collateral material. Make a study of beauty product special offerings in department stores and quality boutiques to get a feel for how the experts of merchandising show large amounts of product in a way that makes buying appealing. Signs are extremely important; their effective use is discussed later.

Image Displays

Although image displays can be highly effective in merchandising products, image displays are of greatest value when you use them to sell services.

Cloak Products and Services with Desirable Symbols and Messages

Image displays endeavor to link products and services with imagery that is compelling and desirable to the consumer. This link gives the product or service the glow of what it is being connected to.

Those who have studied psychology know about Pavlov's dog and about the reality of conditioned response. Our upbringing, education, society, and culture have civilized us. That civilization process includes conditioning us to respond to certain symbols in collective and predictable ways. These symbols are cultural icons, and they carry a lot of baggage with them. Consequently messages that contain these cultural icons evoke predictable responses, generally consistent across the society.

People laugh at certain things; they are inspired by others. People link certain symbols to health, wealth, and happiness. Image display seeks to capitalize on these predictable responses. By cloaking a product or service message with powerful symbols and images, we try to evoke a predictable and powerful emotional response in the viewer. If done properly, this stimulates purchasing. This is largely because people want to exercise their economic prerogative in favor of the image. They want to vote yes.

We have all been in stores of some brilliant practitioners of the art of merchandising with beauty products. One such operation effectively cloaked their products with the theme of helping Third World peoples develop their local agricultural economies. This message touched the

> By linking haircolor with compelling icon images, you can evoke predictable emotional responses that can stimulate impulse purchasing.

human spirit, creating emotional involvement. Another message that was imbedded throughout was preservation of the world and its resources—something else that people felt strongly about. These are big issues that people ordinarily feel powerless to influence. However, through effective merchandising, the stores presented people the opportunity to exercise economic prerogative and vote in favor of these ideas by purchasing the products.

There are many ideas that people will vote in favor of with their pocketbooks: youth, romance, prestige, glamour, success, fortune, and on and on.

DISPLAY SERVICES BY ILLUSTRATING BENEFIT IMAGERY

"How do you display services?" is a question often asked. An example will dramatize how salon services can be displayed to build business. Salons aboard the ocean liners generally have some pretty imaginative ways to stay fully booked throughout the voyage. Recently, one put a display right out in the salon reception area to promote their full-body mud pack treatment.

Visualize what they did. They had a fully reclined esthetics chair overlaid with a big terry cloth spread. Over top of that lay a full sheet of foil. Across the chair's armrests was a plank on top of which sat a large porcelain bowl filled with mud. Stuck into the mud was a paintbrush. Against the backrest of the chair was a dry-mounted poster that was obviously produced by the marketer of the mud. It pictured a fully reclined, slim figured, totally naked lady. Lying on a beautiful white sand beach with the sparkling ocean in the background holding onto a crystal glass of champagne with a million dollar yacht anchored off shore, she was covered from jawline to toe with the mud mask.

The display sold the service. The model with the beautiful figure, the spectacular beach, the yacht, and the champagne evoked powerful thoughts and feelings. There was a lot of emotional and psychological value attached to those icons. The display cloaked the mud treatment with all that imagery. Thanks to the civilization process, people want to vote "yes" to the lifestyles of the rich and famous for themselves!

Suppose the salon had merely mentioned the mud service on the menu without benefit of communicating the powerful imagery through their display. How many of those services do you think they would have sold during the voyage? Perhaps a few. With the display, cruisers were lining up to purchase this service in droves—and, purely on impulse. That is truly remarkable when you consider that it cost over a $100 to get painted with mud, let it harden, and then shower it off. The onboard salon could not shoehorn another person in for the full-body mud treatment room. Now you know the difference between a buying display and an image display.

Ways to Masterfully Display the Exact Image and Message You Want to Communicate

There are four statements you will be making with your displays, and these statements happen automatically. Make sure that you are fully on top of the message you are communicating.

You Make a Fashion Statement

Just as people judge you personally in the first ten seconds of laying eyes on you, so too they judge your entire salon in an instant. Your salon makes an immediate fashion statement by how it is decorated. Glamorous or casual, business or homestyle, young or old, avant-garde or traditional, high-fashion or bread-and-butter—the statement is there. You are a designer. Your challenge is to decide on the clientele you want and then to create a salon decor fashion statement that communicates an image that will attract them.

Your window, reception, consultation area, and station displays are ideal opportunities to communicate the message you want. Decide on the specific fashion statement you want to communicate, and communicate it purposefully!

You Make a Price Value Statement

The props, images, signs, and other tools you use communicate the quality and value of what you offer. There is a market for McDonald's and for Red Lobster and for the 21 Club. Make sure that your display activity is consistent with the value and price message you want to communicate.

You Can Dramatize Benefits

The best displays creatively communicate the benefits afforded by the product or service. With haircolor, benefits like youth, fashion, romance, and sex appeal can be linked directly to your services by selectively choosing the correct design elements. Merely showcasing the product is not nearly as effective as dramatizing emotional value.

You Can Establish Product Relationships

This is especially beneficial when showing how home maintenance products work in combination. Use displays to cross-sell, up-sell, and re-sell. Also, this type of objective can establish brand relationships between the technical haircolor product and the related home maintenance system. Communicate formulation details that show a synergy between the two.

How to Use All the Design Elements That Make Displays Memorable and Effective

Theme

The best displays have a theme. Calendar themes and holidays are the easiest. But you can use any theme your heart desires from 1950s nostalgia to the signs of the zodiac to Old Master artists. Link all the display activity throughout your salon to the same theme for a cohesive impact.

Lighting

Light it like a work of art. Not only must all display cabinets be well lit, but all displays require incandescent or halogen spotlighting to highlight and dramatize key elements.

Design

Design relates to how all the elements in a display are arranged and placed. The pyramid is the most common design arrangement. Other popular arrangements are zigzag, stepped, repetition, and radiation. Eye flow is a top consideration when designing a display. You want to plan the viewer's eye movement so that your display story unfolds.

Background

The background of the display can really help create a sense of place. The wall can be the background, or the background can be completely open space. A semi-open background, one that can be seen over, around, or through, is another option. It allows viewers to see past the display and into the salon when viewed from the street. Window displays in particular offer a lot of creative opportunity when designing the background.

Movement

Incorporating movement in a display dramatically enhances its effectiveness. A video screen, blinking lights, a motorized device, and even windblown effects all create movement and demand eye attention. Some fabrics and materials shimmer in light, creating the illusion of movement. Studies have shown that movement incorporated into a buying display can increase purchasing by over 1,000 percent when compared to the same display without movement.

Color

Naturally, in a haircolor display color ought to be an important component. Just keep in mind that all display elements need to be color coordinated. Dressing up a shop window is not much different than dressing up yourself when it comes to color coordination. Everything must blend and work together. One of the reasons why good displays often incorporate multiple repetitions of the very same poster or bag or other collateral material is to create real cohesion.

Decorative Props

Displays are imbued with imagery by means of decorative props. These are the elements that imply the benefit you want viewers to link to the product or service displayed. Anything from a mink stole to faux pearls are decorative props. Generally the decorative props communicate your theme better than any other element.

Of course the holidays and seasons of the year have their traditional decorations, such as the Halloween pumpkin and Easter Bunny. It is most powerful if you are able to incorporate seasonal props into your display in a way that moves product rather than merely acknowledges the holiday. For example, put a differently colored wig on each of the pumpkins with some clever signage making reference to a Colors of Fall or Harvest Shades promotion.

Structural Props

Structural props hold things up. A draped table is a structural prop. A holder is a structural prop. Mirrors, cases, shelves, and similar elements enable you to lift up the merchandise to eye level where the impact is greatest.

Functional Props

Some items can be incorporated into a display that are both structural and decorative in nature. A vanity to hold products both creates a sense of place and serves a function.

Creativity

With simplicity as the rule, you can decide on one of a variety of elements to give your display design the master's touch. Contemplate what you could do with the effective use of:

- Lines
- Shape
- Size
- Weight
- Contrast
- Harmony

- Color
- Emphasis
- Focus
- Texture
- Balance
- Proportion

Be fresh, surprising, imaginative, unexpected, thought provoking. Engineer a display that makes people want to linger and contemplate. Your image and reputation as a salon will go up. Store traffic will increase. You will charm people into the buying spirit, and you will be rewarded for your efforts with additional purchasing.

How to Use Signs More Effectively

Signage sells. In controlled studies, signage increased sales at the point of purchase by up to 270 percent. Displays, to be most effective, must be accompanied by a sign. The sign communicates the primary benefit or the special offer that is being proposed.

Use Powerful Point-of-Purchase Words

Some words practically create sales. Be sure to incorporate them in all your point-of-sale messages. Some favorites are:

- Free
- Improved
- Try
- Special

- Sale
- Take
- Select
- Proven

- *Guaranteed*
- *Examine*
- *You*
- *Show*
- *Purchase*
- *Preferred*
- *Pick*
- *Experience*

- *Choose*
- *Receive*
- *Discover*
- *Bonus*
- *Sample*
- *Ask*
- *Notice*
- *Easy*

Notice how many of these words have a command element to them. They indicate action; they are insistent and involving. Use command words—the most potent messages you can incorporate into your signs.

Also, a comment on the word *sale*. A common misconception is that *sale* means discount. Don't believe it for a minute! Sale is among the most powerful command words in merchandising. There is hardly another word that will attract more attention in a store. Some consumers just look for the word Sale.

In the dictionary, sale means "The act of selling. A transfer of property for money or credit. A quantity sold. An opportunity to sell something as to hold a sale." Sometimes a sale is a "disposal of goods at a reduced price"—one of the last definitions given. Do not be afraid to use the word sale without feeling the need to discount. The fanciest boutiques in the nation use the word all the time, and you should make it a part of your merchandising vocabulary no matter how fancy your image is!

Utilize All the Forms of Signage You Can

Opportunities abound to increase sales through the use of signs. You can boost purchasing with signs on the outside of the salon that communicate to the passing flow of traffic. You can harvest sales with signage that appears in the window as well as signs and announcements throughout the salon itself.

Remember the old saying "A business with no sign is a sign of no business." How true it is. A variety of sign ideas can underline your haircolor expertise, or, at the very least, put haircolor on the agenda for discussion.

USE THE SANDWICH BOARD SIGN

One idea is a sandwich board sign outside the salon saying "Today's Special—Free—Your Personal Color Analysis–Walk Right In!" (See Figure 7-1.)

That sign will dependably bring in prospects for you. If you are located in any kind of traffic location at all, you can expect two or three walk-ins daily with this kind of announcement. If it costs $200 or $300 to have a nice looking sandwich board sign made, spend the money. In a few months it may get a little dog eared. Buy a new one! You will find

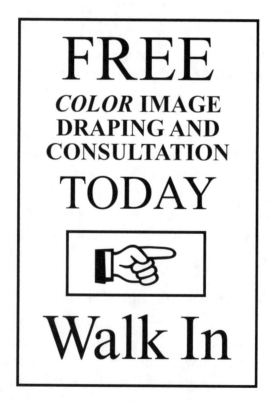

FIGURE 7-1. A sandwich board sign

that this is very low cost-per-fresh-visitor marketing and helps you get more value out of your location. If your image insists on something fancier, try a company that makes granite headstones and see what they can design for you!

DISPLAY YOUR MENU AS A SIGN

Another kind of outside sign you can use is one that illuminates your salon menu. Think of how some restaurants present their menu outside at street level so that passersby can stop and contemplate. It works, and it builds traffic. You might even include a "Take one" holder.

Communicating haircolor as a salon specialty right on your window or door builds interest. So also, there is virtue to the idea of listing the whole variety of color services you offer on your outer window to further emphasize your specialty. Some of the proprietary services you have developed and included in your menu can be featured here. Display hot new looks in the window with exciting proprietary names.

USE "ASK ME ABOUT" SIGNS

Consider opportunities you have within the salon itself—the consultation area, for example. "Ask me about glossing your hair!" is a thought-provoking command sign. (See Figure 7-2.) "Ask me about" signs must pose an intriguing question and arouse curiosity to be most effective. The guests will wonder, "What is glossing?" "Ask me about coloring your hair" is not thought provoking. The guest already knows what coloring is.

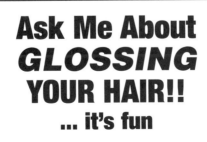

FIGURE 7-2. Ask me about... sign

OUR HAIRCOLOR MONTH PLEDGE TO YOU

During your consultation...
if we forget to tell you
what colors compliment you most
then your haircut
is on the house!

FIGURE 7-3. The promise sign

USE "PROMISE" SIGNS

Another effective sign at the point of consultation is "Our Pledge to You." (See Figure 7-3.) "During haircolor month—Our pledge to you: You will receive a personalized color analysis or your haircut is on the house. Guaranteed!" When the guest sees this kind of signage, they know that you are going to propose something. Furthermore, you have created an atmosphere where that something is automatically okay.

THE CLIENT RETENTION SIGN

The following client retention sign is my personal favorite.

> Dear Guest,
>
> We all agree that a change of style or stylist can be refreshing from time to time. Because we work as a team, it does not matter which designer you would like to try. What we do care about is you and that you continue to visit us so that we can serve you. Feel free to experience the talents of any member of our design team whenever you like.
>
> Very Sincerely,
> Individually signed by each designer

SIGN ALL DISPLAYS

Each and every display—image and buying—must be accompanied by one or more signs if it is to enjoy maximum effectiveness.

Keep in mind that price tags and other product stickers are signs. Shelf talkers, point-of-sale coupons, sweepstakes, and "Take one" and "Try me" offers are all forms of signage too.

USE A VARIETY OF SIGN MEDIA

You also have the option of easels, placards, posters, banners, flags, screens, slides, video messages, holders, or whatever your creative imagination can come up with. Doing something innovative, creative, and surprising with signage is always powerful. Incorporating movement or dimension—even having the sign blow smoke or spray water—will add immeasurably to its effectiveness. Maybe the sign itself can be the message. However, be sure the message does not get lost in your creative designs!

POST ADVERTISING AS A SIGN

You should clearly post any advertising or circulars or other promotional devices you herald through the marketplace. Transform it into a sign on your front door or in your salon window. Have it dry mounted. That way people who have been attracted to your salon by these notices will know that they have come to the right place. You are also announcing to your existing client base the media you use that they can look to for your regular public announcements.

Avoid the Common Signage Mistakes

ALWAYS BE POSITIVE

Never use signage with negative or restrictive messages. These kinds of signs are most often found at the cash out area. "We do not accept checks." "All sales final." "No cash refunds." All these messages must be reworded positively. "Cash, Debit Cards, or MasterCard, Visa, AmEx, and Discover are gladly accepted for your purchases." In fact make sure that you show the credit cards you accept right on your front door. Many people live on these cards, and they like to know right away if you accept them. The same is true now with the popular bank debit cards. Announce the positive option that you accept them.

Instead of "All sales final, no cash refunds" try "Your satisfaction Is guaranteed." Then in a paragraph explain that you will do what you can to resolve any problems by redoing the service if you are to blame or replacing the product if it is defective and accompanied by a sales receipt within so many days of purchase. But word it positively. Never scare away sales with negative or restrictive signs.

Promote Your Offerings Exclusively

Many salons have little signs and displays for all kinds of nonrelated issues. For example, their most valuable impulse purchase area, the front desk, is cluttered with nickel and dime charity collection cans. My advice is to get rid of these immediately. A more successful way to donate to charity is to do a cut-a-thon.

Sometimes the front desk is cluttered with business cards and brochures for home party sales and other gimmicks. Get rid of all that. Many salons put up posters in their window for every event under the sun that passes through town. Instead put a poster or sticker in your window that advertises the product brands available in your retail area. That is a very positive strategy because it can actually help stimulate some walk-in traffic for you. Perhaps another place can be found, visible to all, that can acknowledge worthwhile local promotions/benefits.

The Display Zones in Your Salon and What Works Best for Each

There are four locations that you always want to use for display and that work excellently for haircolor display: the front window, the reception/waiting area, the consultation zone, and the service stations.

The Front Window

The salon windows are an absolute must for display. The front window is the very best place to display haircolor because it can both create a powerful first impression and act as a magnet attracting new salon traffic. Contemplate the benefits of haircolor you could emphasize with an effective exhibit—youth, glamour, sex-appeal, romance, professionalism, leadership. Props, background, and signage are pivotal. Link color services to those appealing values with images that automatically evoke an emotional response.

You should identify a professional window dresser who can creatively carry out your concept. You can find this individual by inquiring at retailers with effective windows like department stores and specialty boutiques. Chances are the person will be a free-lancer. Their fees are often around $100 to $200 to build a window, but some

> Identify a professional window dresser to get your image display activity started. Then, once you have observed the basics, you can assign the task internally.

may work in exchange for your services. They also usually have access to some great props that they can provide on loan. An effective window is among the best $100 to $200 you ever spend on promotion.

Someone in your salon who takes an interest in window dressing can learn all the tricks a professional has to show in about two or three sessions. That person can take over the project from there. You should change your window about every six weeks or up to 10 times a year.

Use the $50 rule: Any extra foils, bags, tissue paper, balloons, streamers, or similar disposables should be obtained for a budget of not more than $50 for each new window campaign. Most props and other fixtures are re-usable. Others can be begged or borrowed from coworkers or even area merchants. You would be amazed at what treasures area merchants will loan in exchange for a little sweet talk and a small sign acknowledging use of a fur coat compliments of the local furrier.

Used mannequins are available, so scour secondhand stores and watch for liquidation auctions of fashion stores. Also your new window dresser partner should be able to get access to great props that were used previously by department stores or other specialty stores. Generally these stores do not repeat decorations from one year to the next and have an inventory that they are willing to sell for pennies on the dollar.

Become a student of window displays by using your own powers of observation; copy what you find effective. An effective window display on a good traffic street or in a plaza or mall will generate ample impulse walk-in business. Plenty of first-time visitors will step into your salon every day based on the attractive power of your window display. Further, it will dramatically boost the profile of your salon in your community. It will add a measure of pride that all the workers and clients will radiate. It can even make new staff recruitment easier.

The Reception Area

The main display in the reception area would be the secondary retail display showing your featured product of the month. Remember, this can be a selection of several items packaged together.

> Avoid the common mistake of giving key display space to close-outs and discontinued retail offerings. Instead, use your prime buying zones to capitalize on your biggest selling offers.

First, feature a single item or package on a display. One element shown in massive abundance is what works. Second, play your strongest cards. Work with proven big sellers. When it is Superbowl time the big grocers haul out the mountains of soda, not the tonic water. Third, keep it neat and clean and well stocked. Make sure that all is in its proper position and that every container is facing the right direction. Let the display look like it has been picked over a little bit, yet keep it fresh looking at the same time.

The biggest mistake salons make with their secondary display is using it to get rid of all the stuff that they are trying to get rid of. Fact is, it still does not sell. All it does is detract from the image of your salon and take away your opportunity to make some real sales with your most powerful offers. This is called opportunity cost. Stuff that does not sell should be given away to charity. An important principle of marketing is to chase your winners and cut your losses.

The Consultation Area

The entry to your consultation zone would be the ideal spot for a major impulse service or feature service display. Remember the one for the full-body mud pack on the cruise ship. If the front area is reserved for retail offerings, then this would be the ideal place for this kind of service display. Any color service that is new or different, any new application procedure, any new series of shades, any new color effect, any new additive or emollient can be dramatized in a display. Remember to include the sign and to add appropriate decorative props that imply vital psychological benefits.

The Service Stations

The immediate areas around the stations where the haircutting and hairstyling, nail art and makeup, facials, and body treatments and services are performed can benefit from display activity. A good idea is to create a shelf or a wall sconce next to each station that can be used to display the featured product package of the month. If it is the haircolor month, then naturally it will be the selection of home maintenance products packaged together for this. Place them on the shelf nicely. Add a little thematic decor to tie it in with the product display in the reception area. Include a sign restating the offer.

Ideally, you want to have a cohesive theme and complementary elements that carry through all your salon displays during a given campaign. The same slogan, the same type-style for the signs, the same colors, the same props, the same overall look. When you make a transition from one campaign to another, you rework all the elements.

CONCLUSION

Display and merchandising is about how you bring your goods and services to market at the point of sale. Haircolor is primarily visual, and so there is tremendous opportunity to build revenues through more effective visual merchandising. Considering that this is a weakness of most salon businesses, extra strong competitive advancement can be achieved by emphasizing this approach.

Merchants of beauty should merchandise beautifully!

Here is what we learned:

1. *We can use both image displays and buying displays to move merchandise, but to stimulate purchasing of color services we must use image displays.*
2. *Our displays automatically communicate messages. It is in our interest to decide consciously what we want to say and then design a display that will get that message across.*
3. *There are countless creative options for displays. It is how we artfully combine them that will ultimately determine the effectiveness of our merchandising.*
4. *Signs at the point of sale have the power to dramatically influence consumer behavior and thus must be included as a vital part of visual strategy.*
5. *The front window, reception area, consultation area, and service stations provide remarkably potent opportunities to communicate strong selling messages through the use of display—the silent salesperson!*

Proven Promotions to Use for Haircolor Income Growth

A dynamic promotion puts haircolor on the top of the agenda for both clients and designers. It provides an opportunity to expand market penetration and income by converting more salon guests to professional haircolor and by upgrading current color clients to more elaborate and expensive color service offerings.

First, regarding discounting as a strategy to attract more haircolor business. Mass-discounting locates the bargain shoppers. And, you can continue to entice these shoppers through continual discount offers. However, it is very difficult to achieve high ticket averages using these promotional methods, and the marketing costs to continually entice these customers become onerous.

Discount strategies may win you customers in the short term, but the long term is suspect. Ultimately, discounting to get people in the door is ill-advised because it may not be possible to retain enough of the bargain hunters at the regular price levels to make the effort worthwhile.

The fact is that haircolor does not need to be discounted to build market penetration and build ticket averages. Consequently, we focus our attention on nondiscount promotional strategies.

In "Proven Promotions to Use for Haircolor Income Growth,"
you learn:
1. the law of promotion
2. the three main haircolor promotions:
    a. the grand opening of your haircolor department.
    b. the haircolor month.
    c. line introductions and extensions.

The Law of Promotion

Take note of the law of promotion: Public promotions succeed more with internal inducements.

It is crucial to imbue all your staff with color consciousness and make sure they are fully onboard with any promotion you unfurl. A good salon manager knows two markets: the public market of clients and potential clients and the internal market of workers and staff. A common mistake is to forget to market ideas internally and only focus the marketing efforts on the public.

It is both unfortunate and common that salon staff are not fully briefed on promotions and offers that are being put forward in salon advertising. Consequently, they are not in a position to be responsive with salon guests when asked point blank questions. There is no excuse for this. Salon team briefings must take place weekly, at the very least, with everybody's presence absolutely mandatory, no exceptions.

"Posting specific financial service goals and results for all salon personnel to view helps everyone clearly see what is expected and what is achievable."

First, everyone needs to be involved and to be in on things. This is a critical part of the planning process. Recent research on what motivates a workforce most puts "feeling in on things" ahead of pay as a motivational factor. Energy is high when everyone takes ownership of an idea or promotion and fully understands the role they must play in the great drama as it unfolds!

A salon management should be open with the staff about the numbers. Let the team see specifically where the performance is and what goals everyone commits to. This idea of keeping financial information from employees is based on fear. Though it is not necessary to disclose all the nuances of margins and profitability, it is important to share information about revenue streams that are being produced, where they are coming from, who is producing them, and where you as a team want to take them. Let everyone see what the starting numbers look like. Organize ideas together to build market penetration and income share. Devise specific plans of action and objectives for each and every participant. Effectively executed, this process builds a lot of excitement and enthusiasm.

Next, formulate an internal reward system. The three main types of rewards are for individual performance, team performance, and salon performance. Put most of the emphasis on rewarding salon performance so that even those who only improve marginally experience the win. Set measurable goals. Track and post progress daily or weekly. Build a lot of recognition around successes. That, in fact, is the number one thing a staff wants—recognition and public appreciation for a job well done. It's how you can create a salon culture.

The Three Main Haircolor Promotions

The three main haircolor promotions are these: the grand opening of your haircolor department, your annual "haircolor month," and your line introduction and seasonal line extension activity. Emphasize these efforts to build your haircolor business. Then, improvise with these ideas and give them new twists and angles over time.

The Grand Opening of Your Haircolor Department

Very few salons have a dedicated haircolor department. Years ago fewer than 5 percent of salons had a dedicated retail area. Most salons have awakened to the reality of profitable product retailing. They have created a product shopping zone within their salons. In the years ahead more and more salons will create a haircolor department. Haircolor will grow into such a profit center that many salons will experience more cash flow from coloring services than from cutting services. Imagine! Ideally you assign square footage in proportion to revenues.

When you create your haircolor department—and the sooner the better—have a massive grand opening celebration. A grand opening celebration of any kind can be your most successful promotion. Next to the opening of a new salon location, there will be no greater opportunity for a large-scale promotion than the grand opening of your haircolor department. That is why you should to move fast while this is still quite newsworthy so that you can attract media coverage to complement your other promotional efforts.

Employ a variety of promotional devices.

Use Outside Signage and Decoration

You could use banners, streamers, lights, and a whole variety of grand opening razzle-dazzle. You can bring in special oversized temporary roadside signage. You may want to have a hot air balloon and bring in a brass band and give away hot dogs! Make it a spectacle.

Neighborhood Direct Mail

This would be a great time to do a general distribution to all qualified residents in your trading area announcing your grand opening and inviting them to some festive gathering.

Here is an idea that may seem radical, but the proof is that it works. This particular technique has worked effectively for other business categories, but it has also proven effective in the salon business. Let's call it the Sample Select Series Sell Grand Opening Promotion.

SAMPLE STRATEGY: Sampling is the most powerful way you can introduce a new product or service to the marketplace. You let people try your offering for free. True, it is the most expensive way to introduce something new. But, it is also the most effective. Sampling enables you to gracefully take advantage of the most powerful offer in marketing, which is to give away something for free with no strings attached.

Naturally you will want to build value first so that the recipient of the free offer feels particularly graced.

Actually, a lot of wise and experienced practitioners of the salon craft believe that you are better off giving something away for free than discounting it. Sampling gives it away for free in a way that can be executed with class.

SELECT STRATEGY: Sampling the entire population is wasteful. You do not want everyone as a client. You cannot serve everyone effectively. Not everyone fits the qualifications of an ideal haircolor client. You do not appeal to all demographic or psychographic categories, and that is perfectly fine. The only consumers you want to sample are your target ideal clientele.

If I could suggest a great demographic it would be female, aged 30 to 50, employed outside of the home, college educated. Now, the psychographic emphasis would be physically active, community involved, socially active people who are out and about publicly. Keep in mind that this is only a suggestion. You need to pursue the clientele with whom you are most comfortable and with whom your own heart rests.

Now the question is "Where are they?"

It is possible to identify them on public mailing lists. You can rent lists of households in your trading area that contain your target population. You need to work with a qualified list broker to help you sort through the possibilities. With a little digging, you can get lists of households in your trading area that contain the specific demographic and psychographic profile you want to target.

Another option is to select specific postal walks that are concentrated with the kind of residents who are your ideal target market. This is not quite as powerful as the mailing list option, but it can work fine. The post office can help you with a map showing how all the neighborhoods are divided up into postal walks. You could

> You choose your clientele. You cannot handle and you do not want everyone as a customer. Focus on the friendly neighborhood residents presold on quality haircolor with the means to pay for it!

actually drive down the streets to eyeball the homes and residents to decide which ones you want to promote to.

SERIES STRATEGY: Having decided on a sampling campaign and deciding on the area residents you are going to target, you next prepare a series of direct mail packages. These distributions will communicate your message to your prospects with the goal of getting them to visit.

There are several items you could include to maximize the effectiveness of your mailings: first, an envelope to contain the items; second, your salon menu; third, a letter; fourth, a gift certificate. Other possibilities include your business card, a haircolor brochure, or a salon newsletter.

The Envelope. The envelope would contain your logo, full return address, and a message. Use an oversized envelope. Research shows that odd-sized envelopes, especially large ones, get opened and read more frequently than regular business-sized envelopes. Make a statement on the outside of the envelope like "Your Special Invitation and Gift Certificate are Enclosed"; "Open at Once ... Your Limited-Time Grand Opening Gift Is Within!"

The Letter. The letter on your letterhead introduces your salon, tells of your grand opening, and shares the good news of the enclosed gift certificate. A half a dozen paragraphs of three or four lines each is all you want. Get to the point quickly and ask for action.

> *Dear Neighbor,*
>
> *You are cordially invited to enjoy a beautiful professional haircolor service! It's yours—compliments of the house— simply by calling 555-1234 and arranging your appointment right now!*
>
> *Actually, it's our way to share the great news of the Grand Opening of our brand new "Beaux Arts Haircolour Salon." It's the very first haircolor specialty department anywhere around, and we thought you would be interested in coming in as our guest.*

> *You are entitled to beautiful, fresh, soft-to-the-touch hair-color. At the "Beaux Arts Haircolour Salon" that is exactly what you can expect. Your color is custom formulated. With the rich conditioning emollients contained in our exclusive line of color, you are guaranteed to experience a rich full color with remarkable shine. Aren't you due for a little pampering right about now?!*
>
> *Your Gift Certificate is enclosed, so you can celebrate our grand opening season in style and with flair. Call the new VIP hotline at 555-1234 and arrange your time right away. We're here right now waiting for you, so call now.*
>
> *Yours,*
> *Beaux Arts*
>
> *P.S. Your enclosed Gift Certificate is exclusively for you. By call-ing 555-1234 right now, you'll receive a beautiful custom hair-color service. It's yours—compliments of the house—during our Grand Opening, so call 555-1234 and arrange your appoint-ment before our celebration is over. Why not do it right now?!*

A few things to note about the letter copy. First, it is client focused. The emphasis is on the benefits the client receives rather than on how great the salon is. Second, notice the extensive use of "you." Third, the letter has emotional content by appealing to luxury, entitle-ment, and even fear of loss. Fourth, the letter contains a P.S. That P.S. is as good as a headline, so it is valid to restate your proposition or primary benefit in the P.S.

The Gift Certificate. The gift certificate would entitle the recipi-ents to a complimentary professional haircolor service as a way to introduce them to your salon. You need to be specific about which color offerings the recipients are entitled to. Generally they will be able to select from a generous but defined group of permanent and semi-permanent options. We personally have had success limiting it to semipermanent options only. It is true that many patrons also select additional services not on their complimentary list.

You should add in fine print the days and times when the certificate is valid. Make it universally valid to maximize response. Give it an expiration date a few weeks hence to prompt a speedy response. You could indicate the requirement to call a specific number and ask for a specific person as your response key. Mention that they must say they will be using their certificate when making their appointment. You should also specify that they must be 18 years or older so that you do not end up with a lot of young daughters whom you would rather not sample.

The Series. As mentioned a series of mailings is involved. Actually, you will mail several times to the very same list of prospects. Each mailing should build on the previous mailing. Ideally, you will be able to remove people from your continuing mailings once they have called to make their appointment. But either way you keep on mailing. Perhaps four or five times to the same list.

Your enclosed letter will change each time. The theme of the second letter may be "We haven't heard from you yet, so pick up the phone and call us right away." The third letter may say "You don't know what you're missing! Listen to what your neighbors are saying. Call now before it's too late." The fourth letter could be the final notice: "We haven't heard from you, and our celebration is just about over. Arrange your time at once." A fifth letter could be the absolutely last chance: "Perhaps you were out of town, but you must make it a top priority to phone right now. We practically have your color here waiting for you to arrive."

Your response may go down with each subsequent mailing, and then you may suddenly get your best response of all. However, as long as you continue to pull a valid response, it makes great sense to continue to work the list. You can only do this grand opening series once, so milk it for all it's worth. Keep in mind that these letters could be two or three weeks apart so you could unfold your entire promotion over a period of 60 to 90 days.

Though there are no specific test results to cite, this same promotional strategy should work for an Anniversary Celebration and as a promotional series to new area move-ins. You can get lists of new area move-ins by paying attention to home sales. These lists are available.

If you have got deep pockets, you can use a different envelope with a different sales message each time. You could vary the inserts—one time a brochure, another the newsletter. You could change the look of the gift certificate or alter the offer slightly. All of these things would need to be tested for effectiveness. Also, you could find that after your second or third mailing, your response drops off too dramatically to continue.

However, on the first and second mailing you should get all the activity you can handle. You could drop 500 or 1,000 to start to gauge response and then stagger additional mail drops consistent with the response you can handle. You will get response!

SELL STRATEGY: If you execute this promotion with success, you will get more samplers than you can handle. Bring each one through your regular consultation. Offer additional services as appropriate: treatments, lash and brow tinting, highlights, textures—it will vary by client. However, make it a definite point to recommend additional service options to each and every one. And, of course, design a complete home maintenance package for each new color guest.

Because they are receiving so much for free and because they are fashion motivated, many of the visitors will have a feeling of obligation and take you up on your extra service and product recommendations. Some salons have found that more than 50 percent of the samplers made additional purchases on their first visit.

> Offering upgraded services to free sample guests will help perfect consultation skills while generating great revenues at the same time.

One thing for sure, if you have a team of designers and colorists that you are turning into a sales force, you will find that this is excellent on-the-job practice with live prospects.

MEDIA RELATIONS

A way to lure color addicts into your salon is through media relations. Do the PR work and get feature story coverage from your local papers and broadcasters. While it still has the shine of newness and newsworthiness, your public relations efforts surrounding the grand opening of your color department should yield fruit. The angle you take is crucial. For example, "A Local Response to a National Trend" would be a great feature idea. Think about "Local Business Evolves to Accommodate Aging Baby Boomers" and "Color Leads Fashion Parade" as other great story hooks.

Start by getting the specific names of all the targeted media personalities in your market. Focus on those most likely to report fashion and features. Radio talk shows and local television talk shows need to be on the list as do all the newspaper, television, and radio feature news desks.

You need to put together an attractive press package with a one-page release, a cover letter, other salon literature, and a before-and-after example or two for the visual media. Send them out. Follow up by phone to make sure that they were received. Quickly review with your contact why their audience would be interested in a story on the topic and why it is relevant and worth covering. Offer to provide additional information. Thank all contacts for the courtesy of their time and consideration and leave it with them.

You may want to consider a press party or a press conference. Put the press on the invitation list for seminars, fashion shows, and other events you produce.

Your best strategy is to have a long-term public relations plan so that you regularly funnel great story ideas to the press. A salon public relations campaign every three or four months is not too often.

We could do a whole section on courting the media, but the most effective ongoing serious strategy is to release seasonal color collections to the press and position yourself and your salon as being the source for coverage on haircolor. Consumers interested in haircolor will read these reports, and many of them will give you a try. There are some excellent books on how to effectively unfurl a successful media relations campaign. Use them as a source for wonderful and effective ideas.

GRAND OPENING ADVERTISING

The new phenomenon in haircolor advertising is the advertorial— an ad that looks like a feature article. This is paid advertising, so you have total control over the message and the call to action. You also have control over placement and run dates. The new twist is that it looks like a regular news story because of its layout, use of photos, captions, screens, typestyles, and headlines.

The advertorial is especially valuable for attracting makeover and serious color clients. It combines high fashion and before-and-after–type photography with loads of compelling copy about the appeal of quality professional color. It has a feature story look, and it reports color fashion using your salon as the primary source of information and opinion. There is a low key call to action at the end of the copy.

This kind of advertising is expensive, but it does magnetize the highest-quality color client visitors through the door dependably. These people are in the market for a makeover! So, even though you may invest over $50 per first-time visitor with this marketing approach, your salon is able to achieve an even loftier average ticket because of the quality of guests attracted.

If you are not able to get a jolt of free publicity from your press campaign, your grand opening is the ideal time to initiate this new-fangled advertising approach.

Another advertorial idea to consider is to have your local paper create a Grand Opening page featuring your new color spa. Your newspaper representative can solicit all your suppliers to take out a congratulatory ad. Naturally the paper will do a meaningful feature on the history and future of haircoloring and your salon as part of the deal.

My personal experience has been that this kind of advertising activity works like magic! I did this kind of a promotion with the grand opening of a retail department at one of my salons. I included a very powerful FREE offer to build traffic, and the salon was busier than a pancake house on a Sunday morning.

> The most powerful offer for haircolor is the FREE professional haircolor service offer.

If I were repeating the effort with the grand opening of a haircolor department, I would offer a FREE color analysis and color draping at the very least. More to the point, be really bold and offer a free professional haircolor service on a no appointment, first come first served basis. You will have people spilled outside the door all day long! It is just a one day event, and it will give the designers plenty of opportunity to consult and up-sell treatments and highlights on live prospects. It is great practice, and it will automatically cause a tremendous amount of awareness about your color department in your community.

Keep in mind that in a grand opening situation you need to set aside a kickoff budget that can range into the thousands depending on the size of your salon and market area. Then for the first year, you will budget perhaps 6 percent of salon revenues for your ongoing campaign. After a year, you can probably move that down closer to the 3 percent range.

THE FOUR CONSISTENCIES OF ADVERTISING

If you are not acknowledging the importance of consistency in your media communications yet, your haircolor grand opening is a great time to start.

Consistency of Location. Once you find productive media, advertise in those sources consistently. Avoid the temptation to dilute your ad budget by spreading your message seed in ten different directions. Yes, at first it is valid to test and track. But once you find acceptable levels of response from particular media outlets, stick with them. That way your audience will know where to find you. For example, one great salon appeared each and every week in the TV section that comes with the weekend newspaper. They have been in that vehicle consistently for ten years, week in and week out. They do not advertise anywhere else except in the Yellow Pages. Their clients and potential guests know where to find them. That is one of the reasons they are on top.

Consistency of Look. All of your general advertising—and all of your printed communications, including all salon resources—must bear your image signature. Logo, typeface, feature model, layout, and other design elements are all candidates for your signature look. The ability to provide the public with a consistent and regular image that builds confidence is one of the great virtues of chain and franchised salon operations. You will want to do the same thing yourself.

Consistency of Message. Know who your audience is. Know the message that appeals to them. Repeat the same message, with minor creative twists, over and over and over again. The bottom line messages are never lost.

Consistency of Repetition. You need to repeat your message over and over again for it to bear fruit. Research indicates that the public only notices about one in six of our promotional communications. Further, they typically have to experience the communication five times for them to make the connection. This means sending out 30 messages to make a dent. So why do so many businesses stop after once or twice claiming no value? For one thing, if the message is weak, there is not much value. But if the message is strong, just the consistency of repetition is lacking. Make your advertising a campaign, not a single shot in the dark!

Post Card to Salon List

Quite naturally you promote your haircolor grand opening to your own salon list—that goes without saying! It is amazing how many salons fail to maintain a mailing list. That is a serious error in business judgment. You should have as large a list as possible. Everyone who has visited your salon should be on the list. It is perfectly fine to have two or more persons in a household on your list and to include all residents in each appropriate mailing.

Actually, the direction to move in is list segmentation. In your universe of salon clients you can have numerous subsets. You can divide them demographically, geographically, by services received, by ticket average, by retail purchases, by source of first business, by whether or not they have ever sent referrals. The segments are endless, and that is why it is vital to obtain all the data you can about salon guests. By segmenting your list, you can really begin to target your promotional dollars to efforts that will yield the most powerful return.

> By segmenting your customer list to reflect current buying patterns, you can focus on creating offers designed to expand your relationship with each client.

For the grand opening of your haircolor department, a promotion that would have many goals, you should mail to your entire list. Are you able to segment your list into categories like the following?

a. Male/Female
b. Never colored/Regularly colored
c. Retail purchaser/Nonretail
d. Age 25–50/Other

If so, you would be able to mix and match categories and target each market segment with an offer that will move them along to greater purchasing.

For example, you could target the 25- to 50-year-old female who has never colored her hair with one offer (e.g., to get her to try haircolor), and the 25- to 50-year-old female who does color her hair but is not a retail purchaser with another offer (e.g., to get her to try retail). Everyone can get the same post card, for example, only the offer on the back changes depending on the market segment they belong to. As you can begin to tell, list segmentation will give all of your promotions much more power.

POSTERS

An underused but potentially highly effective promotional medium is the use of posters on bulletin boards. This is something the independent salon and booth renters can avail themselves of inexpensively. Remember that in this day of beautiful full-color photocopying on oversized sheets, you can create a beautiful master and duplicate only the number you will require cost-effectively.

The grand opening of your haircolor department is an ideal time to start this kind of a campaign, which can be repeated at strategic intervals. You need to begin noticing and developing a list of bulletin board opportunities in your vicinity. Some likely possibilities include:

- Dry cleaners and laundries.
- Supermarkets.
- Churches.
- Community halls.
- Fraternal organizations.
- Health clubs.
- Educational facilities.
- Public buildings.
- Schools and colleges.
- Libraries.

These bulletin boards are a marketplace. People do stop and look. Your cost of exposure is relatively slim when compared to other media. If you found 30 bulletin boards and it cost you $50 to create your announcements, you would have a very cost-effective communication medium that would yield some action. At the very least, it would be one more time you could get your name in front of the public.

You could take it a step further and have tear-off pads created and attached to your poster with some sort of offer. However, keep this simple and look to this strategy as one that will inexpensively build haircolor exposure.

There are other media you could use, such as radio, television, and billboards. I personally have never heard of a salon enjoying spectacular results from radio. Television can work well for family priced salon chains with a large number of locations in the viewing area. The same holds true for billboards.

You only get to do your grand opening once. Keeping in mind the four rules of consistency, plan your multifaceted attack and see it through. If there ever is a time to pull out all the stops, it is during your grand opening.

The Haircolor Month

Your most dependable regular promotion will be the haircolor month. The haircolor month gives you the opportunity to absolutely put haircolor on the top of the agenda. Again, the approach should not be one of discounting. Rather, focus on promotional activity surrounding value-added offers and sampling. Because your haircolor month can easily be your best money-making month of the year, you may want to plan one for both Fall and Spring!

Some promotional features of the haircolor month are discussed next.

AN AUTOMATIC HAIRCOLOR CONSULTATION FOR EACH AND EVERY GUEST

This needs to be an automatic anyway; but under cover of a haircolor month extravaganza, you can freely talk coloring to every single guest without any risk of appearing pushy or offensive. It's all fun, and all the guests are entitled!

You may want to consider a station sign similar to the one shown here.

Our Haircolor Month Pledge to You
You will receive a personalized color consultation during your visit. It's our way to let you know how much we care that you look your very best. If we neglect or forget to provide you this free service, your haircut and style is on the house!

This not only gives you carte blanche, it also makes sure that reluctant designers are on side and participate fully.

A Color-Enriching Shampoo and/or Conditioning Treatment Demonstration

Of course this is a great way to set up the retail purchase. Now that you can custom blend color shampoos, you can even tell an even more exciting story. Do not forget the color-enriching conditioner for the complete home maintenance package.

Naturally, you have to build value around these demonstrations. Add a little showmanship in the blending. Include a little story about how the shampoo and conditioner brighten the client's hair without causing a change of color. Show enthusiasm and give direction about how to repeat the treatment at home and about how stunning it will make the client look. And, of course, post the closing question: "Why don't I custom blend some for you right now so that you can have it at home to use? It's only $10, and because you just use it twice a week, it will last for months. Does that sound fair enough?"

Special Prepackaged Haircolor Home Maintenance Systems That Are Value Priced

You could have one or two haircolor month specials stockpiled in secondary displays in the reception and retail areas. Your distributor should be able to help you with this. Gift-with-purchase offers work great. The appropriate shampoo and conditioner could be shrink-wrapped with a travel size of the bonus item. Another product grouping could include a certificate for the custom blended color shampoo or conditioner.

Always remember to display in abundance. A dozen or two is not satisfactory. Make it ten dozen or twenty dozen! Put the display in the high-traffic zone. Use a sign: Haircolor Month Special Purchase. Light the display warmly from above with halogen or incandescent lighting. Put a ribbon around or a sticker on each package. Add some accessory props like a dry-mounted poster or two. Make it look desirable.

Up-Sell Luck-of-the-Draw Promotions

A rarely used but highly effective promotional tool is the "Everyone's a winner—draw for your prize" event. In your advertising, you proclaim

"We are giving away $10,000 in salon products and services. Come in for your free prize during our haircolor month promotion. Grand prize is . . . ." Keep in mind that you can have a grab bag, a scratch card, a balloon to pop, a fish bowl, or some other similar device to contain the assorted prizes.

> Have a well-planned strategy with premiums and bonuses. Remember the Minnesota Fats principle. Focus on offers that sample products and services. That way you can entice salon guests into more service and product purchases.

Get the guest involved physically for maximum impact. Guests draw for their prize either before their service or after their service. If they draw for their prize before their service, focus the giveaways on:

- free consultations.
- free demonstrations.
- free services.
- gift-with-purchase offers.

Naturally, you want to focus on coloring and upgrade offers. For example, offer a free haircut with any color, or a free treatment with any color, or a free custom blended product with any color, or a free makeup lesson with any color. These offers force a purchase to receive the gift and can work great. Plus, some of them offer additional upgrade and retailing opportunities as well.

Other free offers include simply a free color shampoo treatment and blow dry or a free color consultation. These offers require no purchase for the client to activate, but they funnel them into an automatic presentation or demonstration to which they feel entitled. Remember that you must specify a dollar value with every offer.

Alternatively, guests could select their gift after the service. One possibility here is to offer a discount on their purchase that day. It could be a dollar amount or a percentage. Though not my personal favorite, these offers do get results and can be used to increase purchases when guests realize that they will receive from 10 percent to 100 percent off the final total. They can load right up and think optimistically.

A better approach is gifts that force the guest in one of three directions:

a. Product purchase—a gift-with-purchase offer, making sure that you specify a minimum dollar purchase threshold to qualify for the free gift.

b. Service consultation—a token gift service with the makeup artist or nail artist to force client interaction with those departments to promote impulse purchasing.

c. Another visit—a gift or value that is valid on their next visit as a way to enhance retention of new visitors brought in by your haircolor month promotional activity.

FREE SAMPLE DAYS

This approach can be particularly effective if you receive a lot of walk-in business or have low market-penetration levels for your haircoloring services. The idea is to get a little haircolor on everybody's head with the goal of either upgrading them to a full color service that day or else priming them for the full color sale on their very next visit.

It seems logical to host these events on high-traffic days. Because it is a sample, you do not have to be too extravagant. A few highlights on top or the bangs would be plenty. Do not forget to get male clients involved too. Make it an exciting and energetic day when everyone is just having a lot of fun. This gives the designer ample opportunity to talk about how much fun haircolor is.

Keep in mind the Minnesota Fats principle when doing a free sample day—have your next shot planned. You will want to have two or three special offers prepared, the first would be for the guest who decides to use the occasion to go ahead and enjoy a full haircoloring on the spot. These impulse purchases will happen if you make a strong offer and display a distinctive sign, notice, or hand bill that captivates the client upon walking through the door.

A second offer is for those who make an appointment for a full color service before they leave that day. The third offer is a bounce-back offer for each and every guest who receives a sample but makes no appointment to return. At least the bounce-back offer will give them something to think about. To add extra punch, you may elect to make the bounce-back offer transferable so that it can be passed to a friend, relative, or coworker.

SPECIAL HAIRCOLOR MONTH PACKAGES

We discussed packages at some length earlier when we covered salon menu development. The haircolor month is a great time to unleash your most appealing occasional packages offering multiple services with incentives. Keep in mind the "special of the day" approach that can also work exceedingly well during the high-energy period of a haircolor promotion.

PROMOTE INTERNALLY

Always remember the law of promotion. Get the salon team to start thinking in terms of hitting a home run with each guest during haircolor month (see next page). That will help them hit home runs every day. Think of it this way: The haircut appointment gets them to first base; the treatment sale advances them to second; a permanent or semipermanent color service moves them to third; and bringing the whole look together with foils and highlights gets them home. Then, to really rack up the runs, start thinking of retail products being runners on base. The way to hit a grand slam is to get a service home run with at least three products purchased by the guest. Now you're really ringing the cash register!!

Promote Your Line Introductions and Extensions

When you introduce a new brand of haircoloring, that is a new line. When a manufacturer creates a new package of haircoloring products, that is a new line. When you or a manufacturer releases a new series of colors or design effects to a pre-existing brand, that is a line extension. Some manufacturers produce several lines. They add new color assortments to their existing lines regularly. Line introductions and line extensions happen with haircoloring practically every season. It is fashion. With haircoloring, there is always something new!

Think for a moment of the apparel business. All the big designers produce several lines. Periodically, they introduce a new line. They

LET'S PLAY SALON BALL!

Here are the rules:

Each designer is a team.

Each day is a complete game.

Each salon guest is an inning.

The object of the game is to score as many runs as possible during the game, which lasts one day. Runs are scored by a combination of service sales and retail sales. Each sale advances the prospect for a run based on the following formula.

Service sales. A single salon service is a single hit. Multiple salon services on the same client are for extra bases. Two services is a double, three services is a triple, and four services on the same client is a home run. No service sales is a strikeout.

Retail products sold represent players on base. One product is a runner on first. Two products is a runner on first and second. Three is a runner on first, second, and third. Four products or more is an automatic bonus run. No product sales means no one on base. Alternatively, you could make a $10 retail sale a runner on first, $20 gets runners on first and second, and so on.

Runs are scored by adding the retail sales and service sales results at the end of each client visit. Note that each time you obtain the fourth sale of any combination of products or services you score a run. Each combination of sales beyond four earns you another run. You can receive up to a total of five runs on a single client!

This run chart gives all the possible combinations.

Services	Products	Runs
0	1	0
0	2	0
0	3	0
0	4	1
1	0	0

(continued)

Services	Products	Runs
2	0	0
3	0	0
4	0	1
1	1	0
1	2	0
1	3	1
1	4	2
2	1	0
2	2	1
2	3	2
2	4	3
3	1	1
3	2	2
3	3	3
3	4	4
4	1	2
4	2	3
4	3	4
4	4	5

At the end of the day, each designer adds up the total runs. You can put several designers together on one team if you wish to get a little friendly competition going. But also make the salon one big team striving for a total number of overall runs.

Of course, the salon manager, at his or her discretion, can establish some bonus run categories. A package of services or products could be good for a bonus run or two. Maybe cross-selling a guest into the nail or makeup department can be good for an extra run. You can use your own circumstances and goals to customize the game for your objectives.

Be sure to award prizes. You can reward daily, weekly, and for the full promotion period. You can recognize individual performance, team performance, and salon performance. Everyone wins!

extend their existing lines. This is what all those fashions shows are all about. Typically, when you walk into a department store, you see all the new lines and line extensions out front. Because they are the latest, they get the fresh promotion and best floor space. They are also generally premium priced.

Note also that if a department store were to introduce a new designer to its collection there would be a major promotion. If they decided to add the Ralph Lauren, Calvin Klein, or Tommy Hilfiger line, the introduction would be a really big deal!

We in the salon business must do exactly the same thing. Whenever you introduce a new manufacturer to your collection of haircolor lines, you have got an ideal opportunity to have a promotion. Whenever one of your existing color manufacturers comes out with a new line, you have an outstanding opportunity for a major promotion. Whenever one of your existing lines is extended with a new collection of colors, you have an outstanding opportunity for a major promotion.

Also, you have full opportunity as a designer to create your own seasonal haircolor looks and give them names with market appeal. The only one who says that you cannot do it is you. Do your own models. Take your own photographs and promote your own looks. Why not? When it comes to haircolor, design advanced looks that require two- and three-phase coloring—signature looks with premium price tags that are your design. This is how big money careers are built.

One of the biggest common mistakes salons make is that they fail to promote haircolor line introductions and extensions effectively. Even the big players are typically very weak when it comes to color line introductions and extensions. Commonly, new color lines and seasonal colors are introduced by salons to their clients with a whimper, if at all. This represents a major lost opportunity. Those salons that learn how to introduce and extend lines effectively will secure a very powerful competitive advantage in their marketplace because it is so rarely done well.

"Master the ability to extend your color lines effectively and you will capture a very powerful competitive edge."

There are three central themes to discuss surrounding introduction promotions: color line replacements must be clear-cut; line introductions must be accompanied by a major promotion, ideally with education as the theme; line extensions need to be promoted as premium service offerings.

COLOR LINE REPLACEMENTS MUST BE CLEAR-CUT

Replace haircolor lines by "crossing the Rubicon." One of the common reasons salons introduce a new line is dissatisfaction with their existing line—a perfectly legitimate reason to make a transition. Staying with something that produces embarrassing results simply does not make sense.

Yet, because of the fear associated with changing lines, salons often not only completely neglect the line introduction promotion but, worse, often fail to complete the technical transition. This is such a common problem as to warrant special comment.

Any advancement in our professional or personal lives requires that we confront the unknown and proceed on faith. There is an old saying that if you are not progressing toward your goals, see what you are hanging on to that is holding you back! One of the main reasons salons fail with line introductions is that they spinelessly hold on to the old line—the one with which they are dissatisfied—as a fallback in case they encounter a challenge or puzzle with the new line. So they make no real commitment to change. They do not venture out of their comfort zones. What generally happens is that the salon barely cracks a tube of the new coloring. So rather than force themselves to grow and improve, they end up staying with the same old same old.

It is all about fear—fear of change, fear of making a mistake, fear of not knowing enough, fear of a negative client reaction. If we are to grow personally and professionally, we must confront our fears. And that is why salons must make a Rubicon decision when they replace a line of haircolor. Anything less is simply not adequate and will universally result in failure.

A lesson from history: Julius Caesar and the Roman Legions were returning from triumph in Gaul when they camped at the north side of the Rubicon River just before crossing back into Roman precincts. In their absence Augustus Caesar had captured control of Rome. Envoys were sent to Julius from Augustus to tell Julius to dare not cross the Rubicon lest he and his legions be slaughtered at once. In truth, Julius Caesar's armies were content in the lands north of the Rubicon. After years of pillage and plunder, they were fat and rich and not anxious to fight to recapture Rome.

Julius had a dilemma. Masterfully, he coaxed his Legions over the bridges that crossed the Rubicon. Then, just as Augustus Caesar's armies appeared, Julius ordered that the bridges his Legions had just crossed now be burned behind them. With that bold move of daring and leadership Julius cut off his own Legion's only escape route and forced his armies to stand firm and do battle. And the rest is history as Julius took back his position as Emperor of Rome.

My feeling is that when you introduce a new line to replace an old unsatisfactory line, you must completely rid your salon of the old line immediately. Every last tube and bottle must go. No excuses, no exceptions. You must cut off the escape route. You must burn the bridges behind you and force your salon to master the new line quickly . . . to make your mistakes early . . . to confront your fears while they are still infants . . . to get right back up when you fall down . . . and to advance confidently toward the shining city of artistry and creativity with a dominant command of your haircolor destiny. You must have courage and force yourself through the growth curve!

Only Introduce or Extend Haircolor Lines under the Glorification of a Major Haircolor Promotion

Salon consultants should not waste their time with salons who fail to cooperate with this requirement completely. If a salon will not cross the Rubicon and will not burn their bridges and force themselves to master and dominate the new line, the consultant should move on. If fear governs a salon, it will never get to see Rome.

During the Age of Retail, it was not uncommon for salons to order introductory packages, put the products on the shelf, and then watch them collect dust only to be returned or practically given away.

How many times did people have to go through this routine before finally understanding that if there is no commitment to do what it takes to make a success, there will not be a success!

Part of that commitment means a major one-day promotion that has an afterglow lasting for several weeks. Ideally, the one-day major line kickoff promotion should be the culmination of the education series that introduces the new line technically to the salon's designers.

> Introduce a new color line without the benefit of immediate promotion and it is practically doomed to fail before it even gets started.

Remember the law of promotion—public promotions succeed more with internal inducements. When it comes to any line introduction, the internal inducements start foremost with sessions of intensive technical education.

Technical Education Sessions. It is the responsibility of salon consultants and manufacturer educators to deliver meaningful inducements to get the stylists aboard the educational program. Furthermore, it is the salon owner's and manager's responsibility, in partnership with the product distributor, to provide internal inducements to entice the undivided attention of designers during the line introduction promotional period.

Instill Ownership. Salon managers and distributors absolutely must entice designers into ownership of the line introduction. This process must be started before the line is even introduced. It starts with the distributor's salon consultant bonding with designers and winning their involvement in the decision to replace the old line or introduce the new line. A new color line simply cannot be imposed on someone. Designers have left shops over less! Merely relying on the natural interest, cooperation, and motivation of designers is not going to get the job done. The front line who interacts with the consumer must be completely won over. Failure there will result in the ultimate failure of the line introduction.

Create Recognition. Internal inducement is also accomplished by making the preliminary education process rewarding and involving. Stylists are often independently minded. Demanding their participation in classes can sometimes stir resentment. Better to command their interest and entice their participation through the power of personal influence and mutual respect. These educational sessions must be absolutely exciting and inclusive. The educator must be dynamic and have powerful leadership skills. If recognition can in any way be linked to the educational process, all the better. Further, the education should be repeated on a second and even third occasion in rapid succession. These additional sessions can both review and deliver additional advanced material. Reviewing information frequently stimulates retention and action.

Stage a "Grand Introduction" Day to Kick Off the Consumer Promotion. The big line kickoff day should also be the culmination of the line introduction educational series. A dynamic educator should be in the salon for at least one entire day to demonstrate, lead, and guide. The presence of the guest educator can be the big highlight of the line introduction promotion.

Internal inducement is very important to your new line grand introduction day. One recognition criterion can be based on how many haircolors are applied the day the educator is there. Does the whole team reach a certain goal of color services performed on that day? How many guests are brought in to the haircolor arena for the very first time? How many home maintenance haircolor programs are sold that day? You get the idea. From that Grand Introduction day, you continue the celebration for a period of a few weeks or up to a month.

In preparation for such a day you need to bring to bear the full brunt of point-of-sales promotional techniques including window display and posters and signage throughout the salon. A special edition newsletter to your client list is the best possible way to create excitement. See whether you can get some co-op funds or a quantity of preprinted material to help make your direct mail introduction more successful. All this promotion of your major kickoff day sets the stage for your month-long line introduction campaign.

LINE EXTENSIONS NEED TO BE PROMOTED AS PREMIUM SERVICES

Start seeing line extensions as the promotional opportunities that they are! Think like the fashion store and jump on these opportunities to offer the latest in fashion and design to your clients . . . and naturally encourage them to take immediate advantage of them so that they too can be the first with the latest.

There are several things that you can do to put line extensions on the top of the agenda.

Create a Feature Wall Area Where You Can Display Model Photos That Change with the Seasons. As soon as a new series of color shades is introduced, you will color and style some models, get photographs taken, and redecorate your feature wall. The wall is best placed either in the reception area or adjacent to your haircolor consultation zone.

Make Use of Point-of-Sale Materials Provided by Your Color Manufacturer. These extensions are always accompanied by posters and brochures. Bring them into play. In the last section we discovered how you can use collateral materials when creating image displays for color months and introductions. This display activity will be one of the significant cornerstones of your haircolor promotions. Use display to stimulate interest in and purchasing of your new line introductions and extensions. Further, make sure that literature is presented smartly on the reception desk, in the waiting area, in the change room, and in other high-exposure areas.

Have Everyone Who Works in the Salon Wear One of the New Shades. Be your own live models. To add an extra measure of power, have all designers wear a pin or button describing the color they are wearing: "I'm wearing Auburn Lights" or "I'm Honey Gold."

Bring Your Menu into Play. Make a printed announcement proclaiming your new colors as a special of the day, week, or month and have that attached to your salon menu. This would be one of those great opportunities when designers could embellish their consultations with the special opportunity for guests to receive the very latest fashion shade for a small extra charge. Naturally, you will want to have swatches and other point-of-sale material handy in the consultation area.

CONCLUSION

If you were looking for imaginative ways to promote haircoloring without going the $5 or $10 off coupon routine, you now have plenty. Once you have the grand opening of your haircolor department completed, you can plan for two regular haircolor months annually and from two to four line introductions and extensions each year. Focusing your effort on these opportunities will give you ample opportunity to unfurl four to six haircolor promotions each year, which is plenty. There is no doubt that any of these major promotional opportunities gives you the genuine opportunity to double your haircolor income . . . in 30 days or less!

Here is what we learned:
1. *It is not necessary to use discounting strategies to build haircolor market penetration and service ticket averages.*
2. *The law of promotion means that you use internal inducements to put haircolor on the top of the agenda for all staff members.*
3. *You will want to focus on the three main haircolor promotions: the grand opening of your haircolor department; your haircolor month; and your line introductions and extensions.*

Persuading Guests into Haircoloring

Haircolor is the fastest growing service category for salons. Haircolor sales have had many years of double digit growth. The population is getting older and is looking to haircolor to preserve a youthful, healthy appearance. Fashion magazines and television talk shows have put haircoloring front and center, making coloring more desirable and appealing to consumers than ever. All these factors are working to your advantage. The momentum is there.

It is up to you to take advantage of it. People are converted to salon coloring one at a time. As stated earlier, two major trends are at work. First, the percentage of the population choosing to color their hair will continue to grow. Second, the percentage of those choosing professional color over home color will also continue to grow. These megatrends mean more money for salons poised to profit.

You can look forward to higher income, a more loyal clientele, greater prestige as a designer, and more satisfaction in your career. But where the rubber meets the road is in how you interact and communicate haircolor with each and every guest who visits your salon. Aside from constantly developing your technical knowledge and skills, you must package yourself and personalize your service to achieve major haircolor success.

In "Persuading Guests into Haircoloring," we discover:
1. How to funnel all guests into a haircolor consultation.
2. Ways to make more influential haircolor prescriptions.

3. How to adapt to each client's psychological preferences.

4. Ways to sell multiple color services to the same patron.

5. How to dissolve client resistance and motivate more clients into professional haircoloring.

How to Funnel All Guests into a Haircolor Consultation

Make Sure Everyone Plays Their Part

Create an atmosphere that quietly dissolves the number one reason salon guests hesitate and procrastinate about haircoloring—their fear. The key is to establish a feeling of confidence and security while creating an atmosphere of expertise. These impressions must be conveyed immediately.

Let's quickly review some of the fundamentals.

EVERYONE LOOKS THE PART

Talking haircolor is talking fashion. You must be a fashion role model to clients and provide leadership. That means that you wear color in your hair all the time. You are literally a model for haircolor in your salon.

Make sure that the haircolor style you choose is appropriate for your clientele. Wear coloring in a fashion that will be appealing to salon guests. In addition, always dress up to go to work to maximize your own professional image and enhance client confidence in you.

EVERYONE ACTS THE PART

Behave like a color specialist. That means that you must show supreme confidence in your abilities. If you show doubt in your body language, facial expression, or words, your salon guest will read this. Consequently, your ability to effectively discuss a fashion image that includes color as an accessory will be diminished.

The persona of the colorist is not fully developed in the consciousness of society. People have images of what they think about when you say nail artist, esthetician, makeup artist, hair dresser. The window of opportunity is still open to engineer the most positive perception imaginable for the colorist.

A colorist should be someone who shows leadership. Other characteristics include someone who is fashion forward, is a confident communicator, and has the designer's eye. The colorist is a role model, someone of financial and business success and personal sophistication, a person of human warmth and feeling. You communicate your colorist persona by the very way you carry yourself.

POSITION SOMEONE AS MASTER COLORIST IN THE SALON

This makes real sense, and is especially helpful for salons with designers in the first years of their career. Haicoloring is an art. All the great designers and artists of the ages have served an apprenticeship under a master. So identify a colleague in your salon who can play the role to the hilt. Give this person a real measure of credibility in the eyes of your salon guests. It will help create a sense of ease and confidence for the client.

Make Sure You Communicate Haircoloring Ceaselessly

Up to now we have reviewed more than 100 different things that you can do to proclaim haircolor expertise and pre-eminence. At this point you want to make sure that you are using every trick in the book to communicate haircoloring to the client before the actual consultation even begins.

Make sure visitors see haircolor on the salon sign. Make sure they see haircolor displayed in the window. Make sure they see haircolor mentioned on the door. Make sure they see your most recent newspaper advertorial blown up, dry mounted, and secured on an easel immediately adjacent to the reception desk.

Make sure first-time visitors are given a new client survey when they walk up to the receptionist. In addition to their name and address and other relevant details you can ask questions like these in the following example.

CLIENT QUESTIONNAIRE

Would you like to consider a change of style or color?

Are you wearing color right now?
If yes:
- ❑ Is it a professional formulation or home dye?
- ❑ Are there any challenges you are encountering with your haircolor?

If no:
- ❑ Have you worn it in the past?
- ❑ What did you like most about wearing haircolor?
- ❑ Were there any challenges that you encountered?
- ❑ What would be important to you in wearing color again?

If you have never worn haircolor, why not?

What would be important in deciding to give haircolor a try?

Would you like your color designer to suggest some color and style ideas that would flatter you?

A questionnaire like this is a very powerful way to get clients thinking haircolor. It forces the discussion. If they were not thinking haircolor before they arrived, they are now. Once guests complete the questionnaire and give it to the receptionist, they return to the waiting area. On the table in front of them they see:

- your salon haircolor menu.
- your haircolor benefits brochure.
- your before and after picture books.
- a binder containing article after article from various magazines about the virtues of haircoloring for everyone.

Often, clients ask if they can use the washroom. As they walk down the hall they see numerous snapshots of smiling faces on your color client board. In the privacy of the washroom they learn all about your featured haircolor brand by perusing the manufacturer's point-of-sale literature. Returning to the front, they cannot help but notice all the commotion and excitement and all the people with foil on their heads.

Consider this interesting research. People only comprehend about one in five messages that come their way. They generally have to receive a message six times before they will act on it. This means that you have got to communicate the haircolor message about thirty times to properly stimulate an impulse purchase of something like haircolor. Plan out all these messages intentionally, and work to make them as effective as possible.

Take the New Guest on a Salon Tour

To transmit some more haircolor messages, take your guest on a tour of the salon. Here's a sample of things to point out and say.

> *"Hello, my name is Pat. As you can tell from my name tag, I'm one of the master colorists and style directors here at the salon. Let me take a minute and show you around before we get started."*

"Here is our feature wall with salon models wearing our latest color collection. We really design colors and styles here that are refreshing and quite popular."

"Here are some of the great magazine and news stories that have been printed about our renowned haircolor work. We like to think we have got the best haircolor reputation in town, and that is why so many people are relaxed about having their hair colored here—even if it is their very first time."

"This is where we keep our awards and diplomas for our advanced haircolor education and achievements. We attend all the top color trainings and even bring top color designers and educators into our salon to stay absolutely current with the latest styles and advances in coloring."

"Here is our color and style consultation area. You will be sitting in one of those chairs in just a moment. It is part of our customer service tradition to share the very best ideas on color and style with each individual client. The goal is to help you enjoy a flattering style that shows off your best features."

"Here is our color application area. Practically everyone who visits us wears color. Many of them are trying it for the very first time because they feel comfortable due to our excellent reputation and dependable, consistent, and pleasing results."

"Here is our color formulation area. Everyone is completely comfortable because we use only the latest formulations that are very gentle on the hair and contain rich emollients that actually make your hair look and feel healthier than ever before. You would be amazed at the wonderful potions and treatments you can have that make your hair more beautiful than ever."

"Here is a robe for you to put on in our change room over there. Then just find a comfortable seat in our consultation area over here, and I will meet you there in a couple of

moments. By the way, be sure to turn down your collar because we don't want it exposed lest we drip some color on it
or something."

They step into the change room and receive a powerful barrage
of additional color messages. Perhaps you have wallpapered the change
room with haircolor posters or put in place a sign that guarantees their
satisfaction with your haircolor services.

Next they seat themselves in a consultation chair. Remember, you
want the mirrors strategically located so that they reflect back on the
haircolor application area. Let the guests linger there for a moment or
two uninterrupted so that they can drink in all the fun, excitement, and
showmanship evident in your haircolor application zone.

By having everyone play their part, by relentlessly communicating the haircolor message, and by bringing new guests through a
preplanned tour, you will be able to funnel all guests into a haircolor
consultation.

Ways to Make More Influential Haircolor Prescriptions

"Begin with the end in mind" is a fundamental principle of success that
surely relates to how we communicate with salon guests. Decide first
on the results that you want, and then design your communication
strategy to make it happen.

Consultation is an art. The art of consultation means harmonizing
the client's practical needs and psychological wants with the realities of
nature and current style and design. Doing all this and then motivating
action with grace and style takes skill.

Put Purposes First

The client has motives, and so do you. The client's motives are both
practical and psychological, but mostly psychological. Practically all salon
visitors are dissatisfied with their appearance when they walk through

the door. They want to look better to others and feel better about themselves. Their purpose in visiting is to undergo a pleasing transformation in tune with the image they want.

You respond to this with a motive of your own, the motive of discovery. Because your purpose is to discover areas of discontent and create solutions, encourage guests to elaborate on their problems with their hair and find out the challenges they are encountering with their home maintenance.

The client's psychological state and self-esteem requires sensitivity on our part. It is not unusual for people to bombard themselves with nonstop, hypercritical self-talk about their appearance. That self-talk can make them feel very uncomfortable and inadequate when interacting with others. Paradoxically, it is often those with the most beauty who are hardest on themselves. The bottom line is that most people desire a feeling of comfort, security, self-confidence, and even recognition and prestige from their appearance. People want to feel good about themselves and want to feel that others feel good about them too.

These desires of the clients create a purpose for us—to help the clients feel good about their appearance psychologically. Empathy and understanding with their current dissatisfaction and fear is first. But beyond that it is vital to reassure clients that the products and services being prescribed will deliver immediate benefit and provide longer-term hope.

Notice that our motives flow from the clients' practical and psychological wants. The universal law of success measures our service and delivers abundance, prosperity, and fulfillment in direct proportion to what we give. The clients are not there to serve our financial goals. Yet the greater the service we render to clients, the more our own lives flourish.

> The best opportunity we ever have to stimulate impulse purchasing of salon services and home maintenance systems is the consultation. Purposeful, confident consultations will impact on your income as well as on client satisfaction and retention.

This makes clear what a consultation is not. A consultation is not a brainstorming session or a free association idea exchange. "How about this?" "Have you tried that?" These are not confident or effective ways to advocate specific services or treatments. You are the expert, not the client. Be prepared to step up and advocate a course of action.

Once you are clear on the real purpose of your activity, you can advance toward some situational goals. There are two: (1) to make the clients feel certain that they are the center of attention and that their needs are foremost in our heart; (2) to create the opportunity to stimulate unplanned purchases of services and home maintenance products, specifically haircoloring and haircolor accessories, as a way to uplift the appearance and psychological state of each client.

Be Interested, Not Interesting

The way to provide influential consultations is to be supremely interested in the needs and wants of the guests. They are their own most interesting subject. They are far more into the idea of you being impressed by them than them being impressed by you. They are at the salon to look and feel better and to be the center of attention.

The common mistake some designers make is to try to be impressive to their clients. Shooting from the hip and giving freewheeling advice can be a turnoff. True, you may see exactly what the client needs. But psychologically, it is far better for the client to identify it first. Some clients are too embarrassed to discuss their weaknesses. In those cases, gently introduce the weaknesses into the discussion. Gentleness and grace are essential here because people are often very sensitive about their appearance.

You must establish rapport, first and foremost. There must be a friendly energy flowing between you and the guest. You want the guest to like you and trust you.

How long does it take to build rapport? That depends. A lot of people are open and friendly, and you can build rapport quickly. A few quick questions about work, family, and home will usually get the ball rolling. Be ready with a smile and a laugh. Make direct eye-contact. Be natural. Take it easy and relax.

You cannot control the guest's mood, attitude, or approach to life. Some guests are quiet and introverted. Others can be aloof or imperious. Some put up a wall and are noncommunicative. It will probably take extra time to build rapport with some personality types. Learning how to understand and relate to the differences in people is a study that will continue for your entire career. Over time you will get better and better at charming your guests and getting them to open up more quickly. Your genuine empathy and a willingness to try different communication approaches will get you far.

It Is All in the Questions

The consultation process revolves around having the clients identify their own problems (perhaps with a little gentle prodding) and articulate their own goals (perhaps with the benefit of some subtle suggestions). Then, the designer presents solutions and motivates action.

We get clients to identify their problems and share their image goals by asking questions. In fact these questions are so fundamental to getting the consultation started off properly that they need to be flawlessly prepared and consistently applied.

> **"Consultation questions are so fundamental to stimulating impulse purchasing that they need to be flawlessly prepared and consistently applied."**

Keep in mind that the questioning process begins with the new client survey. That kind of a survey is extremely valuable because it helps cut to the chase on haircoloring. Without a survey like that a lot of designers find themselves babbling before they get down to what they really want to talk about. The conversation just wanders when stylists do not know how to make tactful suggestions and clients are not aware of their options.

In contrast to that, your goal is a structured consultation that takes only a few minutes and presents multiple impulse purchase opportunities. The clients will know how they responded on your questionnaire and will be awaiting your input during the consultation. This becomes especially strong when you have their completed questionnaire in hand or on a clipboard.

Consider that two sales can be completed before the consultation even begins: the treatment sale and the cut and style sale.

Have an order pad in hand just like a restaurant waiter so that you can take note of the services as they are being confirmed. One column to list the services and another to list the prices. You could also have a section on the ticket for your home maintenance recommendations.

CONFIRM THE CUT AND STYLE ORDER QUICKLY

Here's how much time to spend on the haircut portion of the consultation: *"Janet, when you came in today you were planning on having your hair cut and styled, is that right?"* Ninety-nine percent will agree, and you make note of it on your ticket. That's it. Do not let the consultation get bogged down in a discussion of the haircut. The client has already bought the haircut. This is the time to emphasize the impulse purchase ideas.

The great mistake 90 percent of hair dressers make is that their consultations amount to no more than a discussion of hair length about the ears and down the back and the length of the bangs. That is why they suffer from dreadfully low ticket averages.

When the client is in process, you can talk about the details of the haircut. If the client shows you a picture of a haircut say, *"Great, let me make a note of that for you"* and move on. The picture can actually help you with the color sale if it shows color, so keep that in mind. *"It's not just the cut . . . it's the color and highlights that make the look so great."*

QUICKLY SELL THE TREATMENT

Back to the consultation—still that phase before the consultation. Now is the time to prescribe the appropriate treatment.

Start by identifying the problem. *"Janet, before we get into the specifics of discussing the look, let's take care of any problems you're encountering with the condition of your hair. If you had a magic wand and could change anything about your hair—how it performs, the challenges you encounter with it some days—what would it be?"* That is a nice open-ended question.

When fishing for problems, it is better to ask questions that take a paragraph to answer, rather than ones that require a simple yes or no. If the question is: "Is your hair dry?" and the response is "No," how do you proceed without contradicting her and potentially making her feel foolish?

Janet is going to mention one of about eight different problems that are the most common. Dry hair, static electricity, split ends, flat hair, dull hair, will not hold a style, oily scalp, dandruff, hair loss. You know the list. You hear it every day.

If the guest is a little tongue-tied, prompt to identify the hair problem by using the "How do you feel about that?" questioning technique. *"I see that nature is thinning out your growth on top a little. How do you feel about that?"* Or, *"I see that the environment has left some telltale residue on your hair that is preventing your natural shine from coming through and is making your hair dull. How do you feel about that?"* Or, *"I notice the electricity in the air is wreaking havoc with the manageability of your hair. How do you feel about that?"* You get the idea.

The secret is to word the problem in a way that makes the client the victim rather than the cause. This is important. So, if you see the problem the client is not identifying, use the "How do you feel about that?"

Once the problem is identified, move into a preliminary close. Try the "If I could . . . , would you . . . ?" question: *"Janet, if I could do something here today that would solve that dry hair problem, would you like to give it a try?"* Generally the response will be a firm "Yes" or "I don't know, what do you suggest?" In either event you are now able to fully delve into your specific treatment prescription.

Start your prescription process by including the client's opinion in the diagnosis: *"Janet, based on what you're telling me, and confirmed by my own observation as a professional stylist, you're suffering from* [problem] *and need our* [solution] *treatment."*

Next, use your salon menu as a sales tool. In your salon menu you have specific treatments prepackaged to treat each of the major hair problems that salon guests encounter. So pull out the menu and point out the specific treatment. Be sure to read aloud the two- or three-sentence benefit-oriented copy that accompanies it. The client will be able to see the price.

Conclude this interaction by making note of what you have pre-scribed. *"Let me make a note of this treatment on your consultation record."* Then write the name of the prescribed treatment on your consultation pad. That's it. You do not ask for the sale. You just write it down. You will see that we are going to secure all the sales at once at the end.

Your consultation will automatically be more influential if you focus on the client by planning your questions to advance targeted services.

How to Adapt to Each Client's Psychological Preferences

Refine Your Questioning Strategy

A large percentage of salon guests will indicate on your questionnaire that they would be happy to consider a change, and that they would like your opinion. So at this juncture you take out the questionnaire and glance at it quickly. Think of how the doctor glances at your med-ical history before proceeding with the examination. This is all part of showmanship. The client will know what they wrote on your question-naire. They will be awaiting your thoughts and opinions.

A rule of thumb in any kind of sales is that the person asking the questions is the one who controls the situation. So proceed with more questions before speaking up and making a design diagnosis.

Here is a good question to start with: *"So that I can suggest some-thing ideal for your lifestyle, tell me about the times when good looking hair is important to you. Is it for your career? Is it social?"*

A good follow-up question is: *"Tell me about the upcoming events or activities where you want to look your absolute best. Business functions? Social functions? How is your love life?"*

Another good question is *"How do you want to present yourself? How do you want people to respond to you? How do you want to feel about yourself?"*

These are very powerful questions. The key is to get beyond what clients want. See whether you can find out why they want it. They want to look nice—why??? Who do they want to impress? How do they want to feel about themselves? What are they trying to accomplish?

You Are Selling a Psychological Service

The why factor gets to the psychological aspect of coloring service. Hair can make people feel more confident at school or work . . . feel more acceptable to their friends, coworkers, and aquaintenances . . . feel more romantically desirable. That is why they are at your salon!

Who, what, where, when, and how questions can help reveal the why. Asking these questions effectively will automatically create a more intimate understanding between you and the guest. Encourage your clients to reveal themselves to you. If you find out why your guest wants to look good, you will be able to render greater service.

The bottom line is to get the discussion beyond the hair itself. Get into the feelings they want to experience. There is a psychological pay-off that they really want. That is what they will spend their money on. Reassuring clients that they will receive the psychological payoff creates a make-over opportunity along with the kind of spending that accompanies it.

All this is as fundamental as a doctor asking "Where does it hurt?" In the beauty business, we deal with people's self-image. For us to do our very best work, it is essential that we understand how our clients feel. Where is their self-image hurting?!

Haircolor makes people feel better about themselves and feel better about the image they are presenting to the world. Haircolor is the medicine! Haircolor helps people reflect their personality and individuality. Haircolor is the tonic! Haircolor is a psychological dynamo. And it is not the haircolor itself . . . it is what the haircolor does psychologically.

Haircolor helps people feel better about themselves and express their individuality and ideal image. You are offering a very personal service, and it is important to know what the client wants! Here are some words that can describe the sorts of psychological payoffs your clients desire.

- Youthful
- Healthy
- Glamourous
- Prestigious
- Vital
- Confident
- Wealthy
- Professional
- Leadership
- Sex appeal
- Romantic
- Successful
- Recognized
- Accepted
- Peaceful
- Elegant
- Fashionable
- Respected
- Admired
- Appreciated
- Powerful
- Stylish
- Classy
- Feminine
- Masculine
- Attractive
- Desirable
- Competitive
- Appealing
- Important
- Lovable
- Strong
- Virile
- Fit
- Motivated
- Purposeful
- Cultivated
- Energetic
- Thin
- Worthy

The list is as endless and as individual as each salon guest.

Here is the point to remember. You are not offering clients haircolor. You are offering them the image they want; haircolor is the means by which you design that image. To make haircolor irresistible to your clients, you must link performing the haircolor service to the clients getting what they want and assuring them that the psychological payoff is at hand.

Make Sure Your Stage is Set

Once the client has unloaded, now it is your time to make your design diagnosis. This is where the effort put forth to establish credibility and create confidence pays you back 100-fold. All of that staging makes your recommendations irresistibly influential. You have a lot of momentum on your side at this point. You have a guest who has revealed her self-image problem(s) and who wants the relief you can provide.

If the momentum is not there, it is because there was a flaw in your approach up to this point. If there is resistance or anything less than full openness, it is because you have not set the stage properly. More often than not, if there is any weakness at this pivotal juncture it is that you have not established credibility and confidence. You must exude total credibility and confidence. The biggest social mavens . . . the wealthiest patrons . . . they will all melt if you express charm, grace, composure, professionalism, and credibility!

Personality and attitude make the difference. Magnify those aspects of your natural personality that lend themselves to creating confidence in others. Also, you must rule out fear. You cannot be afraid of the customer. You must not think that the customer is either above you or below you. You must keep your own thinking and attitude positive, clear, and focused.

Ways to Sell Multiple Color Services to the Same Patron

Prescribe Specific Services and Emphasize Emotional Appeal

Prescribe your suggested services with as few words as necessary. Do not sell. Prescribe. "What do you think, hair-doctor?" should be the only thought on your client's mind. You want an atmosphere and psychology at this point where the client is practically on the edge of her chair waiting for your brilliant design vision to spill forth.

Of course, you suggest haircoloring almost always. It is the color that makes the look. One experienced colorist recently reported that about 95 percent of women and about 40 percent of men are appropriate candidates for professional color. Few first time guests will bring up the idea of haircoloring on their own. Yes, they are interested, but they are waiting for you to bring it up. So speak openly and freely. In fact, unless your client is very slow to read the situation, she is expecting a haircolor diagnosis. Everything that you have done up to this point compels haircolor.

Consider that you have already planted dozens of haircolor messages. Your client has probably already formulated pro-haircolor thoughts in her own mind. In the change room, the thought "This place sure does a lot of haircolor . . . if I was ever going to try it, this would be the place" probably swept across her consciousness. As she sat unattended in the consultation chair for a few moments watching all the color being applied, she must have thought, "Gee, that looks fun— I wonder if they will recommend it for me too!"

Now, prescribe three or four coloring services. Link the psychological payoff the guest wants to the coloring services you prescribe. Each client will receive a permanent or semipermanent coloring. Each will receive some highlighting service. Each will receive a final glossing treatment. Many will receive textures. Many will receive lash and eyebrow tinting. With some, you will color the beard!

> **"Before the consultation begins, you want to set the stage so that new guests automatically say to themselves, *'This place sure does a lot of haircolor . . . if I was ever going to try color this would be the place.'"***

Have your salon menu in hand so that you can show the guest the specific offerings you are prescribing. Immediately start out with benefit statements. Bring forth the exact psychological graces for which the guest has disclosed a desire.

"Jennifer, to keep you looking youthful and to stay competitive on your career path, we'll start with this particular demi-permanent color service. Here it is in the menu. It says . . . ."

Do not ask for confirmation or comment. Simply make note of your prescription on your order pad. She will be able to see the price in the menu. If a little clarification is needed, you say something like *"I think you hair falls into the mid-length range,"* and she can see what that means from an economic perspective.

You continue: *"Now, to add a little electricity to your love life and send out the right signals to eligible bachelors, we'll perform the foil service called . . . . But let's just do the top third of your head. Here it is in the menu. It says . . . ."*

Again, do not ask for confirmation or comment. Simply make note of your prescription on your order pad. She will see the price in the menu. You have already given her the price clarification.

You continue: *"You want your hair to have a real healthy glow, so it is vital and natural looking. We will complete the hair design with the . . . glossing, which will even everything out and bring your whole look together. Here it is in the menu. Now, you really have such a beautiful skin tone, but it could be so much more flattering and sexy by showing a little contrast, so we will tint your eyebrows and you will be a show stopper."*

Four color services now. You are getting ready to close the sale, and have not even talked shade. Imagine! Nor have you gone into any details about chemistry or technique beyond what may have been alluded to in the menu copy. The usual recommendation is to make the sale at this point and worry about the details like the shade later. Or, if the client wants to go into the details, use the details to close the sale. But that's getting ahead of ourselves.

Securing the Transaction

KNOW WHEN TO CLOSE

You close when the guest is ready to buy. Learn to recognize when people have psychologically bought. The moment they mentally own, experience, or possess what you are offering, they have bought. Watch for body language signals and language clues. The twinkle of the eye, the hand to the chin, the sigh, the relaxation of the shoulders are all physical buying signals. Any language that indicates ownership or possession is a buying signal. When the grammar and word choice make the subtle transition from the possibility of owning to the experience of owning, you can tell that they psychologically own what you are offering.

This is one of the reasons why you want to make your service presentations consistent and well practiced. If you can focus your own attention on the psychological dynamic and be sensitive to the state of the client, your closing percentage will skyrocket.

PRESUME THE SALE

Having prescribed the four color treatments, stand next to your guest —not in front, not in back, but next to. You both look at the list of services you have written down. Of course, next to each service you have indicated the price. You quickly review all the services you are going to be performing as benefit statements: *"We'll make your hair softer and more appealing to the touch with the . . . treatment. Then, . . . for career power and prestige, . . . for romance and desirability, . . . for your fashionable and glamorous image. For a stunning final touch, we'll tint your eyebrows. With the cut I have in mind, you'll walk out of here looking like a million dollars. Now I need you to join me over here where we will start phase one."*

The best way to close is to presume the sale and make a simple direction for the guest to follow. When she gets out of the consultation chair to follow you, she has bought everything. That is the smoothest approach I know—it is how you presume the sale.

CLOSE WITH A MAGIC PHRASE

You can also close the sale with a magic phrase. Here are two great ones: *"Does that sound fair enough?" "Would you like to give it a try?"*

"Mrs. Client, I don't mind telling you that I would really enjoy doing this for you. And we can do everything while you're here today. We'll have you on your way looking great and feeling fantastic within 90 minutes. Does that sound fair enough?"

"Mrs. Client, I don't mind telling you that I would really enjoy doing this for you. We can do everything while you're here today. We'll have you on your way looking great and feeling fantastic within 90 minutes. Would you like to give it a try?"

It is our social custom that the vendor asks the consumer for permission to proceed. This is part of the role we play as professionals. You communicate to the guest that you would like to do it. You let the guest know there is time on the schedule to do it. Then you use the magic phrase. It is that simple.

You will be amazed to find out how many say yes. Those magic phrases really advance your cause. They are low-key, nonpushy ways of indicating to your clients that they have the opportunity to proceed while gently encouraging them to do so. You are appealing to their sense of fairness. You are indicating that haircolor is something that you try, like a new food, and that the consequences are nothing to fear. Does that sound fair enough?

Be Sensitive about Price Disclosure

Now a word about price disclosure. First, as we learned earlier, prices are specifically printed in the menu. In instances where there are multiple prices for the same service, make it clear to the guest which price applies by casually mentioning the price division that is hers. Mention short hair or long hair, full head of highlights or a third of a head of highlights, your status as a master colorist or a color technician. Whatever the price division is, simply mention the category that applies to her and she can see the price implications in the menu. Also, she has seen the price for each service that you have indicated on the prescription pad. You have disclosed price.

Though you may have a Total line at the bottom of the prescription ticket, you need not total it at this point. As a waiter does in a restaurant, you leave it open in the event additional items are added before the visit is concluded.

Some prefer to show the guest the grand total figure at this time to avoid any potential for question at check out. My personal opinion is that there has been adequate price disclosure and there is no need to draw more attention to the price unless the client specifically asks.

Conclude your consultation by giving the guest specific directions as to what to do next. Summon her from the consultation area. This is a very important junction. If there is going to be a question or an objection, this is when it will most likely come out. Let's discuss some of the major issues that can emerge at this point.

QUESTIONS ARE BUYING SIGNALS

Always remember that questions are buying signals, not to be seen as challenges or conflict. If there was not any interest, there would not be a question.

Remember the principle that the one asking the questions is the one in control of the conversation. So when you receive a question, respond with a question. Usually you will respond with a question asking for clarification. With a little finesse, you will be able to use these questions as the bridge to the sale.

For example, the guest may ask you questions or want you to elaborate on possible shades. This is easy. Say, *"Well, let's decide on that right now."* Bring out the swatches and books and get the client physically involved in the selection process. All you ever have to do is use the alternative option close. *"Jennifer, I myself could go with either choice. Which do you prefer?"* That is a closing question—called the alternative choice close. When she states her preference, she has bought. Once she has bought, stop talking and start the service!

> **"Questions do not mean challenge or conflict. Questions are a good sign because they are buying signals! If there was not any interest, there would not be a question."**

The same basic approach applies if the guest wants to detail the cut during the consultation. *"It might be kind of fun to go with bangs, or we could wisp it over to the side . . . that might be more business-like. Which do you prefer?"* Her preference statement is a statement of purchase.

The instant clients buy you give directions as to what happens next. You need not ask if they have bought, or if they would like to buy. Simply presume the transaction. By following your instructions, they communicate their purchase.

How to Dissolve Client Resistance and Motivate More Clients into Professional Haircoloring

Sometimes you will get an outright objection. You can close the sale on the strength of your response to the objection. Use the reason the guest gives for not proceeding as exactly the reason why they should proceed.

Isolate the Real Objection

First, realize that there are two kinds of objections: sincere objections and insincere objections. It is a waste of time responding to insincere objections. You want to identify and eliminate insincere objections so that you can respond to the real issues standing in the way of advancing.

The first way to eliminate insincere objections is to simply ignore them. Make a rule that you do not respond to an objection unless you hear it said at least twice. You ignore it the first time you hear it because it is generally just idle chatter. Do not validate it with a response. If the guest mouths the same objection a second time, you can answer it. Ignore all objections on the first go around.

The next way to determine whether an objection is sincere or not is to isolate it. Insincere objections are not easy to isolate because a person does not want to commit to something that is not real. The way you isolate any objection is with the "other than that" question: "Other than [the objection], is there any other potential reason for hesitating?" If she gives four or five other reasons, you can be sure that most of them are not sincere. Sometimes people are just too embarrassed to tell you the real reason why they are reluctant to proceed, and so they come up with a whole tangle of justifications.

Sometimes you just have to move on because of time issues. So realize that if you are not able to isolate a sincere objection, it is not likely that you will close the sale promptly without the aid of advanced selling and communication strategies that are beyond the scope of this book.

Become a Master of the "Feel, Felt, Found" Response System

The response to sincere objections is easy because you only have to remember three words. The three words are "feel, felt, found". Once you have isolated the objection, show empathy for the client's feelings. *"Jennifer, I understand how you **feel**."* Next, indicate that you have heard this concern before. *"Other people have sat in this chair and **felt** that way at first too."* Then you give your response. *"This is what they **found**."*

Now you provide turnaround evidence. Types of evidence you can bring to bear include facts, statistics, new developments, special ingredients, advanced techniques, and testimonials. Here's an example: *"Jennifer, I understand how you **feel** about the potential of color fading. Other people have sat in this chair and **felt** that way at first too. This is what they **found**. The new advanced conditioning sealers that we use here will lock the color molecule right into the hair shaft so that it cannot wash out."*

Next, relate the evidence to the client: *"The reason I mention this is because you want bright exciting hair that makes that power statement for you at work."*

Next, bridge to the close: *"Once our clients recognize that they can depend on our advanced color techniques, they have the confidence to go ahead and proceed. Does that sound fair enough? Great, please follow me to the application area so that we can get started."*

> *This is an important formula. So to summarize:*
> 1. *Start with the "feel, felt, found" formula.*
> 2. *Provide turnaround evidence, which is some fact or testimonial that dissolves the guest's concern.*
> 3. *Relate the evidence to the guest personally and psychologically.*
> 4. *Bridge to the close. Use a magic phrase. Give a specific direction. Does that sound fair enough?*

Suggest More Haircolor as a Way to Overcome Objections

Often responding to an objection opens the door to an additional sale, an additional service, or a home maintenance product. You can use objections as an opportunity to upgrade. *"Jennifer, I understand how you **feel** about regrowth. Other people have sat in this chair and **felt** that way at first too. This is what they **found**. By adding some foils, you are able to achieve a lot more dimension to your look, so a little regrowth can actually give your hair the appearance of more depth and fullness."*

Next, relate the evidence to the client: *"The reason I mention this is because you want dynamic hair without worry."*

Next, bridge to the close: *"Because our clients recognize this added value, they have made foiling our most popular color technique. And for your hair, you will want this particular foiling service. Here it is in the menu. You will want all your hair highlighted. Now you have got a design with a lot of class and a lot of staying power. Does that sound fair enough? Great, please follow me to the application area so we can get started."*

Know How to Handle Price Objections

When you show your prescription pad list of the half-dozen services you are proposing, you can expect a few patrons to swallow hard. That is only natural. You are prescribing a makeover caliber of service that could run well over $100. Typically the client will ask you whether or not it is essential for her to have everything done. She is hoping that you will back down on a service or two so that she does not have to spend as much and can still get the same thing.

Hold your ground.

Try to get the price objection specified down to one or two services. Maybe, for example, it is the $70 highlighting service. Once the objection is isolated, an effective strategy is to put the decision on that service off into a secondary time frame later in the visit. *"Jennifer, we're not going to be getting to the highlights for about 20 minutes. Let's go ahead and get everything else started. When it comes time for the highlights, I will let you know. Think about it between now and then. At that time, if you choose to go ahead and do this for yourself, we will do them. If not, we won't. Does that sound fair enough?"*

Most will say, "fine" and you will have just closed all the other sales.

Now, over the next 20 minutes the only thing Jennifer is thinking about is those highlights and whether or not she will give herself permission to do it. It will be the only thing on her mind. When it is time to apply the highlights you say, *"This is the time. I think we should do it. They are the key to the sex appeal of the whole look. What do you say . . . shall we give it a try?"* You will get one of three responses:

1. Many will say, "yes," and you proceed at once. No additional talking is necessary. Avoid talking yourself out of a sale.

2. Some will respond with an outright "No." Accept the verdict. Perhaps you can plant the seed and say "Well, think about it for the next time."

3. Some will express uncertainty. These folks really want to say, "Yes." They simply require a little validation and reassurance. So, do not back down. You could say, *"Oh c'mon! You're going to look and feel like a million dollars when we're done. You deserve it. Let's go ahead and give it a try!"*

In these instances, you have to take the sale. *"Here, come with me back to the application area."* You may even reach out and put a couple of fingers behind her elbow and give a gentle tug.

It is a good idea to have a trump card left in your hand at this impulse sale juncture: *"Jennifer, the reason why I insisted on the highlights as part of this design is the striping effect. I took into account your whole body and physical presence and just knew that the slimming, thinning, and slenderizing effect that the highlights give to the complete look would be something that you would really appreciate. These highlights are going to slim your appearance right down. Give it a try and see for yourself."*

Practice Your Responses to the Three Big Fears

People decide to start coloring their hair purely for emotional reasons. So, too, emotions convert people from home coloring to professional haircoloring. What are these client emotions, and how do we care for them? What psychology will inspire clients to try salon haircoloring? Understanding these issues better will enable you to massage some very important messages into our consultation communication.

There are four great human motivators, the psychological dynamo propelling behavior and activity:

- Fear
- Greed
- Guilt
- Exclusivity

Two of these motivators in particular come into play with haircolor: fear and exclusivity.

The greatest motivator of all is fear. But with haircolor, fear is a two-sided coin: on one side, fears opposing haircolor; on the other, fears compelling the haircolor solution. It seems there are three main fears opposing haircolor. Let's consider them along with potential communication strategies for responding to them.

FEAR: AM I WASTING MONEY?!

Many consumers do not yet see enough added value from having it done in the salon and do not want to wind-up kicking themselves for blowing money on something they could just as easily have done at home. How do you respond to this?

First, a lot of the work done at home has to be adjusted in the salon. This winds up costing more money (and time) to correct than if the person had it done in the salon to begin with. This is a point to emphasize to anyone who comes to you for a color correction. Try to persuade them not to experiment at home coloring in the future. Next time maybe you will not be able to fix it! Also, it can be useful to mention an unfortunate episode or two to influence any new color clients to stay away from trying to color their hair at home.

Second, the fact is that a lot of home jobs simply are not good. Does the client feel good about walking around in public with hair that looks a little strange? And, if it does not look odd, does it do the client justice? Doesn't hair that is not quite right create unbearable self-image and self-talk gloominess? Isn't feeling good about ourselves worth something? If all it takes is a few dollars to make someone feel better about themselves in this world, isn't it worth it?

Expanding on this point, the more and better work done in the salon, the greater the contrast will be when compared to home color jobs. As the general public grows more sophisticated, home jobs will simply be inadequate. It is similar to how home haircutting became backward when compared with skilled salon service. People who cared at all about their appearance were compelled into the salon to quash feelings of inadequacy.

Other points that can be made include the fact that carpet, clothing, and towels are often stained at home. This has a cost. Plus, the home color is not free. A package costs $5 or $10 so how much are they really saving when they factor that in?

Also, how about the value of leisure time? People value their free time. Spending an evening in the bathroom fooling around with hair-color is not a joy for a lot of people. It is stressful. There is anxiety. There is a lot of waiting and confinement. That is diminished quality of life when compared to the ease and pampering of the salon experience. Aren't they worth a little treat—a little minivacation in the salon?

FEAR: HOW MUCH ONGOING EFFORT IS THIS GOING TO TAKE?

Fear of regrowth, fear of fading, fear of hair damage, concern about having to be continually in the salon—these can be genuine concerns, especially for first time color clients.

First, consider what the client is trying to accomplish—generally youth and some control over their appearance. Keep in mind that well-designed haircolor and highlights can have a very slimming and thinning effect on how a person looks. Now consider the alternatives. How much time would they have to spend at the health club every day? Talk about a time commitment! And how about the misery and denial of pleasure surrounding dieting? Compare that to the relaxation and pampering of the salon! Is there any comparison? Compared to the alternatives, haircolor is effortless. Unlike exercise and dieting, with haircolor their results are assured!

Second, your custom color formulations coupled with the quality of the product you use actually enhance the condition and appearance of the hair. Furthermore, concern about roots and fading make it all the more important that you suggest highlights over the semipermanent or permanent color. They give the hair added dimension and depth and prevent potential anxiety if the clients' schedule means that the length between visits is occasionally a little longer than usual. Notice again how the solution to client fear is more color!!

FEAR: AM I GOING TO FEEL GOOD ABOUT HOW I LOOK?

Clients want color that reflects their personality and advances their aspirations. Truth be told, many are afraid about how others are going to react to their new color and how it makes them look! They are afraid of negative comments, afraid of rejection. They are concerned about losing position and status within the tribe. These fears can come into play with any makeover-type service.

The first issue is whether they are satisfied with the way they look right now! The answer will be "No, not completely." When you find out why, you will discover that it is fear of aging, fear of losing control, fear of not being okay or acceptable, fear of losing the affections of a loved one, fear of not being able to compete effectively in a youth ori-ented culture! It is all fear!

The solution to the problem is haircolor. Your strategy is to dis-solve any fears associated with the proposed enhancements. Naturally, your reassurance is crucial. First, you could underplay the amount of change they will experience. Describe that you are adding shine and dimension to the hair. You are simply making their existing color bolder and more intense. You might mention that people will wonder whether they just came back from a vacation, they look so relaxed and re-energized.

A second strategy is to help them experience in advance the ben-efits they want from the haircolor. Tell them that others will see them in a more favorable light. For example, the gentleman does not need to fear that others will laugh and call him dainty. Rather, he will appear stronger, more masculine, and virile. He will recapture youth and will look more athletic as well as express a romantic flair. That is what he wants to hear!

Declare that with your haircolor clients will be more successful, popular, acknowledged, appreciated, and recognized. They will look more confident, self-assured, in control, powerful, and happy. Put them in the picture. Let them experience with sight, sound, and touch how well received they are with their enhanced color. Tell them the positive and supportive comments people will be making. Share with them the cultivated, refined, prestigious, well-tailored, classy, elegant, and fashionable image they will be putting forward. Let them know that the color will put a spring in their step and a gleam in their eye!

Color will help them express their individuality and will enable them to more effectively control the response their appearance gets from others. Color will make them more popular, more acceptable, more admired, and more loved. The response they get from others will be exactly the response they want to get. Color will get the job done!

There is an old saying that the sale does not begin until the prospect says no. By understanding the real issues that are at play and by preparing yourself in advance with with effective responses, you will be able to dissolve a lot of resistance and motivate more people into professional haircoloring.

Some Final Thoughts

Anything worth doing well is worth doing poorly at first. Banish fear and discouragement from your mind. Every day you will get better at your consultations and your design techniques as long as you do not give up. Continually strive to improve.

Keep the SWSWSWN formula in mind when you consult: "Some will. Some won't. So what? Next!" Do not let the reality that some are going to decline the haircolor opportunity hold you back one bit from suggesting it to each and every guest with enthusiasm. When someone declines, gently ask yourself, "What could I have done or what could I have said that might have yielded a different outcome?" Then adjust your approach as required and try again with the next one.

The good news is that there is always a next one—and, in the salon, they tend to come along frequently. By being painstaking and fearless about practicing your lines and refining your approach, you will make continual improvements. Ultimately you will get into a zone of awareness and influence that will enable you to entice virtually all guests into professional haircoloring. Look to the near-term day where the one who elects not to have haircolor will be the exception.

Remember, your interest is in the "some who will." Avoid letting the "some who won't" frighten you from offering coloring to the some who will. Remain focused, positive, and stay gathered together for the long march. Have the courage to shake off a "no" response and move on immediately. Focus on the joy and transformation you will bring to the many who will accept your offer. Affirm the merit of your personal goals and desires so that these also sustain you.

Resolve in advance to maintain the psychological equilibrium that progress demands. Take responsibility for maintaining a positive mental attitude toward yourself and others and enjoy the journey. Happiness is the progressive realization of a worthy goal or ideal. What you are about is worthwhile—keep that forefront in your mind.

You are in the midst of the biggest salon service boom in decades—haircolor. Do not pass on the opportunity to offer your clients greater satisfaction and yourself a higher income at the same time! Put haircolor on the agenda. Talk about it openly and watch your prestige and client retention rates skyrocket!

Conclusion

When communicating with people on an emotional level, we have a responsibility to encourage them to do what is going to be best for them. The most successful designers are able to inspire clients to move past their comfort zone into greater aliveness. That means confronting fears and compelling positive change.

Our overall strategy is to minimize the fears that hold people back and maximize the benefits that will propel them forward. Add a dash of exclusivity and you have all the psychological motivation necessary to get the job done.

The trend of more haircolor in the population coupled with more of the population coloring their hair in the salon is the best news imaginable. We accelerate these fashion currents daily through effective consultation. But most importantly, we extend the gift of helping people transform themselves and lead fuller, richer, and more joyous lives. That is the color we add to their lives!

Here is what we learned:
1. *With preplanning, you can funnel all guests into a haircolor consultation.*
2. *By emphasizing the client, your haircolor prescriptions will automatically be more influential.*
3. *Your questions and personality enable you to adapt to each client's psychological preferences.*
4. *You can use a consultation approach that entices a patron to experience multiple color services.*
5. *Practice in advance what you plan to do and say to dissolve client resistance and motivate more clients into professional haircoloring.*

Pursuing Color Clientele

O ne of the benefits of haircolor is that it is the great loyalty service. The goal is to retain as many color clients as possible. They are the most valuable customers you will have, so the more your salon clientele is made up of color clients, the more money you will make.

It is one thing to entice a guest into the haircolor arena the first time. A little effective persuasion can get anyone to try something once. The real value to the relationship comes with the three *R*s: Retaining the haircolor client, referral cultivation, and retail purchasing. Actually the three *R*s work hand in hand and are all crucial ingredients of pursuing the most lucrative color clientele. Furthermore, the three *R*s are all fundamental elements of salon success, whether you are a color specialist or not. And whether it be athletics or the salon career, perfecting the fundamentals is a sure formula for achievement. Practicing and refining fundamentals never goes out of style. Here you will find a few new twists as well.

In "Pursuing Color Clientele," you discover:
1. *the most effective way to retain more haircolor clients.*
2. *how to generate more haircolor referrals than ever before.*
3. *how to maximize retail sales to haircolor clients.*

The Most Effective Way to Retain More Haircolor Clients

Thank you cards, follow-up phone calls, and reminder notices are all effective methods for retaining clients in general. Pre-selling a series of visits via a service contract or voucher book is even more effective and high powered. But absolutely nothing works better than simply pre-booking clients before they leave the salon. With concerted effort, you can get a rather large percentage of color clients to prebook their next visit.

A Power Book Is Built on Prebooking

Ever wonder how some salon professionals become completely booked weeks in advance? Some designers experience such high de-mand for their services that they force new appointment seekers onto waiting lists to be called in the unlikely event of an opening. That is power! That is a power book! That is a cash cow!

How do they do it? They prebook today's clients for their next appointment before they leave. It is that simple!

Prebooking the next appointment is the very first clientele building strategy we were ever taught. Yet how many of us do it without fail? One of the fundamentals of commerce is that we do not get paid for what we know—we only get paid for what we do!

Prebooking Paradise

Prebooking accomplishes several important goals. First, it retains clients for the next visit. Second, it shortens the time between visits. Third, it increases the annual spending value of a client by perhaps 20 percent or more. All are worthy goals.

Set the stage for the prebook. Make conversation about the series of cuts or treatments or color overlays that will be necessary to achieve the look or desired result. Emphasize the importance of discipline and timing in the process.

Casually mention that people calling in at the last minute are often disappointed because high demand leaves no openings. Reinforce the value of convenience for them by arranging for their next appointment now. Fear of loss and a feeling of exclusivity are the emotions to be emphasized. Consistently include these ideas in your discussions, espe-cially with the first-time visitor.

An additional strategy is to prepare a simple notice that is handed to guests at some junction in the service process . . . perhaps when color is processing or they are under the dryer. (See the sample announcement.)

> *Give yourself the confidence and guarantee for yourself the quality service you deserve. Arrange for your next visit today and be assured of the date, time, and designer of your choice. That way you will be secure knowing that your hair will be maintained and you will be looking great all the time.*

Also, you could post this announcement as a sign in the change room, washroom, and at the reception desk. You could paste it to the cover of magazines and styling books.

These communication strategies are designed to prepare the client for the idea of prebooking. That way, when you directly propose the idea, they will have already become familiar with it.

Prebook During the Service

Attempting to schedule the next appointment as an afterthought when the guest is on the way out the door does not work. Too often you wind up in a situation where the guest is in a rush to leave. On the way out the door, she will promise to call for the next appointment. If this is a first-time client, the odds of visiting again have just been re-duced meaningfully. A departure without prebooking works against the worthy goals of guaranteed retention, shorter time between visits, and greater purchasing over the course of the year.

As part of your customer service system, decide on a specific time during the service when you will attempt the prebook. Approach the topic casually: *"Jennifer, I see that you are in here on a Thursday evening. Are Thursday evenings generally a good time for you to be at the salon?"*

After a general confirmation on the time and day that are best for the guest, proceed to explain the reason for prebooking. *"Jennifer, the reason I was asking about your schedule is that we are going to need to*

*have you back in three weeks to move into the next phase of this design
and refresh your color. I will go ahead and schedule your next appointment
for that Thursday at 7:00 P.M. Does that sound fair enough?"*

Notice how we tell the guest what we propose to do and then
ask for confirmation. We do not seek permission by asking, "May I
schedule an appointment?" Asking for permission results in a lot more
negative replies. Proposing an appointment is much more consultive
and professional.

Confirm the Appointment

The first time to confirm the appointment is at cash-out. Write it down
on an appointment card and hand it to the guest confirming the date
and time of her next visit. In some instances you may be scheduling
appointments six to eight weeks out. In these cases especially it is not a
bad idea to send a reminder card. Have the postcard arrive at the
client's address five to seven days before the scheduled service. "We
are looking forward to seeing you. We have got some great new ideas
for you."

When you send out these cards, some folks may call to cancel.
Transform that cancellation call into a rescheduled appointment: *"I'm
sorry you cannot make it then. Thanks for calling so that we can give that
time to someone else. When would be a more convenient time for you to
come in, Saturday or an evening next week?"*

Another strategy is to make confirmation calls the day before the
visit. If you notice a no-show factor coming into play at all, you need to
start confirming appointments at once. Nothing can be more disheart-
ening than the foil highlights you have built your afternoon around not
showing up and leaving a big hole in your schedule. Forewarned is
forearmed. The confirmation call is to communicate, "We have got
your special time arranged for tomorrow afternoon, and we are all
looking forward to your visit."

A talented front desk person may even try to up-sell the appointment on the phone by noting the weekly or monthly special offer.

Do Not Scare Customers Away

You want people to feel free and easy about prebooking. A sign at the front desk threatening to charge customers who do not keep appointments can scare people away. First of all, charging no-shows is a delicate situation to begin with. Though there are times when it is appropriate, especially for repeat offenders, you do not need to shove the policy down everybody's throat with a threatening sign. Second, a newer client who for some reason does miss an appointment is apt to remember the sign, which could easily discourage that person from returning for fear of being charged for the missed appointment.

If appropriate, try a sign similar to this:

> *As a courtesy, we simply ask for a day's notice when cancelling and rescheduling appointments. Thanks for your cooperation.*

You could have the same kind of message printed on the appointment card.

So now you know the secret of creating a fully booked schedule all day every day well in advance. Doctors, dentists, chiropractors, and cosmetologists who are on the ball have known the magic of prebooking and the benefits it provides. Naturally, knowledge acted upon creates results. The principle of prebooking is a fundamental strategy for clientele building. Make sure you practice the fundamentals because they never go out of style!

How to Generate More Haircolor Referrals Than Ever Before

Word-of-mouth advertising is almost a cliché in the salon profession. When clients talk you up to their friends, you are sure to get a progression of new guests in your chair. And the fact is that they are already believers. They have already fallen in love with your work and have that measure of confidence that only personal referral can create.

Leave all this to chance, and chances are you will be left out. Something as important as stimulating referral activity demands a well thought-out plan and consistent application.

Successful proprietors are able to attract several thousand referrals a year by mastering the fundamentals of referral marketing. They practice referral marketing with consistency and excellence. If you can achieve merely a fraction of these results, consider what an impact it would make for you financially. Here are some proven ideas to make it happen.

If at First You Don't Succeed—You Don't Succeed

Cultivate referrals on the guest's first visit. On the first visit, you will probably achieve the most dramatic transformation the client has had in some time. That is when the comments by friends, family, and associates will fly. The client's hair, being a new focus of attention, gives the client an easy opening to mention how great you are and what a wonderful place she has discovered.

Warm up clients fast and early. Lead the conversation with first-time clients in a way that allows you to mention referrals often. If they themselves were referred, then be sure to make a big deal about it. Always talk about how you are getting so busy that you are only able to accept new guests that are referred. Have a complete array of happy stories to share about extended networks of family, friends, and work colleagues who come to you. Make it seem very natural that people are always sending their friends to you. Steadily mention the idea that pretty much everyone new who comes to you is by referral.

Ask for referrals at the styling station. The time to start soliciting referrals is while the guest is still in your chair. Have a planned moment and have specific statements. Be consistent.

For example, your time could be just after you use your hand mirror to show the entire style to your appreciative client. The client nods in approval. You put the mirror down, reposition the chair, look the client straight in the eye, and say, *"You are going to get a lot of comments on this when you return to work and see your friends. You wear the style so well. May I ask a favor of you?"*

Wait for the answer, which is nearly always affirmative. Continue: *"Most of the new guests who come to me do so because they have seen my work on someone who really shows it off, like you. This is what I would like to ask: Over the next week or two, when people mention how great your hair looks, would you tell them where you had it done?"*

Again, clients will almost always respond affirmatively. Then say, *"I have got something for you up at the front desk to show my appreciation. After you get yourself situated in the change room, I will meet you up there."*

Remember, this conversation takes place with the client in the chair before the cape is removed! You are assured to have their undivided attention and agreement at this time.

Introducing Your Referral Program

Intercept your client before she gets to the cash register. Ideally, you will have some paperwork you can provide the client to pass along. This is where a salon menu or image brochure is most valuable. At the very least you must have a business card and preferably a referral card for this specific purpose.

A separate, simple announcement explaining your referral program is also in order. There are a variety of ways these packages can be assembled effectively. For example, one very successful salon assembles three menus with cards attached and three haircolor brochures along with an announcement sheet and a big paper clip holding everything together.

Make an offer to the client rather than to the referral. It is more effective to reward the person providing the referrals with a bonus rather than discounting the first-time guest. Say, *"I would like to give you a $10 or $20 gift certificate [or whatever your bonus offer is] as a way to say thank you for helping to spread the word. Here are three salon menu's and brochures for your purse or keep them in your car. Have them handy so that when friends mention how marvelous your hair looks you can give them one and tell them about the new color salon you discovered. My card is attached to each menu. Tell them when they come in to mention your name on the new client questionnaire they will be completing.*

I will keep track of it for you. You will get a bonus for each person who visits for a service. I will see that it is mailed to you. Does that sound fair enough? Great! Well it seems we both have a powerful interest in making sure your new style looks fantastic every day. Here's the liquid mousse I was telling you about."

Notice how the referral discussion can bridge seamlessly into the retail service.

There is an old Zen saying: "To know and not to do is not yet to know." Everyone will agree that word of mouth is our most powerful form of advertising. An informal survey found that less than 2 percent of clients are asked to send referrals. When was the last time you asked a visitor to send referrals?

If you are leaving it up to chance, then you are being left out! Cultivate opportunities with first-time visitors especially. Refine your referral discussions so that you can drop them smoothly into your conversations. Ask for referrals while you are still in complete control and the client is in your chair. Have a specific referral program with attractive printed matter. Reward those who spread the word. Use your system consistently!

How to Maximize Retail Sales to Haircolor Clients

Point-of-sale displays, mass merchandising, menu descriptions, manufacturer collateral material, and other window dressing help create client awareness and build desire for your home maintenance product offerings.

However, if there is one thing we have learned about impulse purchasing in the salon business, it is that clients will buy your beauty potions on the strength of your recommendation more than anything else. You have got to make an unequivocal recommendation and design a system of products for each salon guest.

Let's talk retailing as it relates to haircolor.

Begin at the Beginning

Just as you merchandise haircolor throughout the salon to impart 20 or 30 subtle hints, so too you need to unfurl the very same strategies with your retail offerings.

Have a retail section in your salon menu that emphasizes professional recommendation. Many salons have gotten into custom formulation of home maintenance products. Some major manufacturers have designed custom formulation systems with haircolor. This all lends itself to a lot of captivating copy. Color enriched shampoos and conditioners are now on the market. These can be highlighted. Naturally the color care and maintenance shampoos and conditioners put forth by every manufacturer under the sun need mention. Special glosses and shiners and fixatives of every discretion can embolden the drama of haircolor. You could go as far as developing a special product menu—just as some restaurants have a wine list or dessert menu.

The order pad you use for capturing your service recommendations can be designed to include space for home care products as well. It is positive to mention home maintenance during the consultation: *"Jennifer, as we are together this afternoon, I am going to demonstrate some techniques and potions that we use here for you to also use at home. That way you have the confidence of being able to step out in style and be recognized for your fashion, glamour, and good looks every day. Does that sound fair enough?"*

During the consultation, you will find that home maintenance product knowledge will enable you to address a number of the fears and concerns surrounding haircolor. A lot of the fears surrounding dryness, condition, breakage, or fading can be addressed by adding home use products to the sale.

Demonstrate as You Go

Each and every time a product is brought into play, you demonstrate it. Remember the value of showmanship. Tell a little story about each product. Get a little involvement going. Tell the client to smell it. Have her touch the consistency. Have her feel the tingle. Make it fun.

At the back bar, tell her specifically about the shampoo, conditioner, and whatever else you are using. Specifically mention the brand name and item name. Describe what you are doing, pointing out any special procedures. Mention why you have selected this product for her and what benefits she will experience with it. Mention how she needs the product at home and how and when she would use it at home.

"Lay back Jennifer, you are in for a treat. I will be using this particular shampoo. It is the best deep cleaning shampoo I know of. Doesn't that have a stimulating, invigorating aroma? Your hair will be free of all the sticky, gummy residue caused by the gels and sprays you use. You need a bottle of this at home to use once a week before your weekly deep conditioning treatment."

"Jennifer, watch how I custom blend for you some special color enriched shampoo with that beautiful color infused right into it for you. It is rich. You will like how your haircolor looks instantly refreshed every time you use it at home. A 12 oz. bottle is only $12 and it will last you six weeks or more. Let me blend one for you right now while all the ingredients are right in front of us. Fair enough?"

At the station, do the same thing. Tell the client specifically what you are using. Specifically mention the brand name and item name. Describe what you are doing, pointing out any special procedures. Mention why you have selected this product and what you will accomplish with it. You mention the need for the product at home and then demonstrate how to use it.

Another time-proven strategy is to put the product container right in the client's hand.

Discuss Other Products That Are Appropriate

Not every product you recommend is used on a given visit. Make time to talk about those that are not used. The expression *"I'm going to get some of that for you before you leave,"* plants a seed. The client will remember what you were talking about when you say that. In fact, at the end of the visit, it will be on her mind to ask about the item before you forget your promise.

One of the reasons people like that expression so much is that it is a little bit confusing. The listener is not quite sure, but thinks that maybe you might be offering something for free. Of course you are not, but the mere possibility of that dependably creates attention and interest.

Design the System

The ideal bridge to the retail service is the referral program that was just discussed. Remember, say something like, "Well, it seems we both have a powerful interest in making sure your new style looks fantastic every day. Here is the liquid mousse I was telling you about."

Now you take items from the retail display and put them on the counter for cash out. Consider these four laws of retailing.

THE LAW OF CONSISTENCY

Everyone is offered the retail service. No matter how busy you are, everyone gets the benefit of it. And, never prejudge if someone is inclined to or able to afford it. You will find that the more they spend on service, the more they will spend on product.

THE LAW OF ONE LINE

You design a home maintenance system by suggesting an assortment of items from a single retail line. People believe lines are designed with products that chemically complement one another. People often feel they sacrifice quality if they mix and match. See how this law is never violated when designing a skin care regime. Abide by it when designing a color care regime too.

THE LAW OF LARGE SIZES

Especially on daily use products, be sure to offer your clients the best value. People generally associate larger sizes with lower costing. Especially if your retail products are big name national brands, you can definitely move clients into family sizes for more economical use.

THE LAW OF LARGE NUMBERS

Suggest the entire array of products that would be appropriate for the client to use at home. Put a whole system together. Think of what they do for skin care in the department store. Do the same thing with hair care. Give your clients the benefit of all the bells and whistles.

Secure the Transaction

You will have a system of a half dozen recommended home use items on the counter. Quickly review: *"Janet, here are the daily use shampoo with infused color and your daily conditioner. Use your deep cleansing shampoo just before your semi-weekly deep conditioning moisturizing treatment. Here is your color mousse for before you blow dry, here is your super hold spray for your finished style, and here is your gloss for those times when you want that extra sparkle and shine."*

Now close the sale. One way to close is to address the receptionist and say, *"Sue, could you reach down and get a bag for this?"* Alternatively, you could say, *"Here, let me get a bag for all this."* These approaches are where you presume the transaction—the smoothest and easiest way to proceed.

You will discover that a noticeable percentage will go right along and take what you have recommended. There will be another group who will want to talk about it for a minute before deciding how to proceed. They might ask some questions. Remember, questions are buying signals.

It may be appropriate for you to whittle down the system in size and number of items. That is fine. Once adjusted, summarize what you have done and conclude by saying, *"These four items are really the cornerstone of your home maintenance system. You will have the security and confidence of guaranteeing that your color will last beautifully for you. Does that sound fair enough?"*

Once you ask the magic question *"Does that sound fair enough?"*, remain quiet, gaze warmly into the eyes of your client, nod your head ever so slightly, silently say "yes, yes, yes" in your mind, and wait for the client's response. If it takes her 20 or 30 seconds to contemplate the purchase, let her have that luxury. Do not interrupt, do not say a word. Affirm the sale silently.

If another round of whittling is required, go through the same procedure.

Finally, you can always have a deal sweetener up your sleeve to clinch the sale: *"I have a little unopened vial of the gloss. Because this is the first time I have colored your hair, you go ahead and obtain your home maintenance program and let me include the gloss as a free 'thank you' bonus. Does that sound fair enough?"*

It works!

Conclusion

Practicing the fundamentals with excellence, imagination, and consistency is the key to color client pursuit. The lifetime value of the color client is substantial. Be attentive to the finer points discussed here and you will not be able to handle the ever growing demand for you.

By pursuing the three *Rs*—retention, referral, and retail—you will have clients pursuing you!

> *Here is what we discovered:*
> 1. *The most effective way to retain more haircolor clients is to prebook them.*
> 2. *You can generate abundant haircolor referrals by developing an upgraded referral program and implementing it consistently with each new guest.*
> 3. *You maximize retail sales by designing a home maintenance system for each salon guest and adhering to the four laws of retailing.*